STAY

FERTILE

LONGER

EVERYTHING YOU NEED TO KNOW
TO GET PREGNANT NOW—OR WHENEVER
YOU'RE READY

STAY
FERTILE
LONGER

MARY KITTEL

MEDICAL ADVISOR:
DEBORAH METZGER, M.D., PH.D.

RODALE

© 2004 by Rodale Inc.

Printed in the United States of America
Rodale Inc. makes every effort to use acid-free ∞, recycled paper ♻ .

"Quick Reference: What Women Need Before and During Pregnancy" on page 64 is adapted from the Dietary Reference Intake, © 2001 by the National Academy of Sciences and reprinted with permission from National Academy Press, Washington, D.C.

The Natural Family Planning Chart on page 186 is used with permission of the Institute for Reproductive Health, Georgetown University.

Contributing Writers: Sidney Stevens, Joely Johnson
Book Designer: Tara Long
Illustrator: Phil Guzy

Library of Congress Cataloging-in-Publication Data

Kittel, Mary S.
   Stay fertile longer : everything you need to know to get pregnant now—or whenever you're ready / Mary Kittel ; medical advisor: Deborah Metzger.
      p.   cm.
   Includes index.
   ISBN 1–59486–053–X paperback
   1. Conception—Popular works.   2. Fertility, Human—Popular works.   3. Infertility, Female—Popular works.   I. Metzger, Deborah A.   II. Title.
   RG133.K54   2004
   618.1'7806—dc22   2004010820

Distributed to the trade by Holtzbrinck Publishers

2   4   6   8   10   9   7   5   3   1   paperback

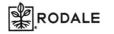

RODALE

WE **INSPIRE** AND **ENABLE** PEOPLE TO IMPROVE
THEIR LIVES AND THE WORLD AROUND THEM

FOR MORE OF OUR PRODUCTS
WWW.RODALESTORE.COM
(800) 848-4735

Contents

PART ONE

OPTIMUM FERTILITY

1

Healthy Women Are Fertile Women

Degrees. Meaningful work. Adventure. A soul mate. Expense accounts. A good breast pump. We are women of the 21st century, and we want it all. Why shouldn't we? Our foremothers shook the foundations of science, politics, and cultural traditions to obtain the electrifying array of options we now embrace. Life expectancy for women has increased by 30 years over the last century—so we have more time to fill the political offices, executive boards, Olympic team positions, religious leadership roles, and military posts that are now our brass rings to claim. Furthermore, "the widespread availability of contraception that first became available to the baby boomer generation empowers us to choose when and if we want to become a mother," observes women's studies scholar Sara Evans, Ph.D., Distinguished McKnight University Professor in the department of history at the University of Minnesota in Minneapolis, and author of *Tidal Wave: How Women Changed America at Century's End.*

As our vision of what constitutes a full life broadens, so does our to-do list. According to the U.S. Census Bureau, more women are waiting longer before they get married. We are spending more time being educated before plunging into the work world. For a growing population of women, childbearing also comes later in the sequence of life events. Twenty-five years ago, only 5 percent of U.S. women had their first child at the age of 30 or older. By the year 2000, one out of four births were to first-time moms in their thirties or beyond.

"Divorce and remarriage and the evolving concept of family are also important motivations for later childbearing," Dr. Evans points out. People may have already had children when they were younger but may strongly wish to have children in new partnerships. The growing number of over-30 mothers also includes single women who have decided not to wait any longer for a lifelong mate, as well as lesbian mothers who are taking advantage of the advances in sperm donation and fertility drugs.

Twice as many women ages 35 to 39 gave birth in 2000 compared to 1978, while the number of births to women ages 40 to 44 more than doubled over the past 2 decades. But as commonplace as it has become, giving birth at the age of 35 or older is actually considered "delayed" or "older" childbearing in the medical books. That's not because 35+ women aren't zesty or have necessarily reached even half of their life expectancy, but because statistically they've moved out of the peak period of fertility when conceiving comes quicker and high-risk pregnancies are less common. "No doctor will disagree that biologically, the early twenties are the optimal time to conceive. But *situationally*, the best time may be much later for today's woman," points out Vanessa Cullins, M.D., vice president of medical affairs at Planned Parenthood Federation of America in New York City.

"Throughout the world, we see a pattern where as a country gets more technically advanced, women tend to delay childbearing as they increase their education and employment status in the interest of providing the best for their children. That's what happened in the United States, and it's also starting to happen in developing countries like Bangladesh and Nepal," says Dr. Cullins.

In addition to the women's revolution and the technological boom weighing in on the age of childbearing, it's become downright fashionable to be a mature mom. Our superstars are looking more capable and beautiful than ever with a baby in tow, including Geena Davis (first-time mom at age 46), Madonna (second-time mom at 41), Kim Basinger (gave birth at 44), and Susan Sarandon (who had babies at 39, 42, and 45). Former *cover* girls now focused on their *baby* girls (and boys) include over-40 moms Christie Brinkley, Iman, and Cheryl Tiegs (mother of twins at 52 who used a surrogate to carry the babies, although the eggs were her own). Going by the pages of the fashion or news magazines, our cultural icons are making later-age pregnancy look glamorous. Even easy.

In truth, delayed childbearing challenges us to become increasingly careful about the choices we make, particularly the ones regarding how well we take care of ourselves over the years. "If you expect to conceive at a later age, it's all the more motivation to be aggressive about preventing premature aging, chronic medical conditions, and reproductive health threats," says reproductive endocrinologist and gynecologic surgeon Deborah Metzger, M.D., Ph.D., medical director of Helena Women's Health in San Jose, California, and medical advisor to this book.

HOW LONG CAN YOU STAY FERTILE?

In 2001, the American Society for Reproductive Medicine (ASRM) launched a public service campaign to get the word out about threats to fertility. As part of the campaign, the slightly disconcerting image of a baby bottle in the shape of an hourglass was posted on buses in major U.S. cities and distributed in flyers to college students across the country. Underneath, a slogan read: "Advancing Age Decreases Your Ability to Have Children."

The campaign is both sobering and encouraging. The first take-home message about age and fertility is that reproduction does not come with a contract for unlimited hours. Eventually all women go through menopause, which means you've had your final menstrual period and thus your last chance to naturally ovulate an egg that could become your genetic offspring, says Michael Soules, M.D., professor of obstetrics and gynecology at the University of Washington in Seattle, who is leading the ASRM infertility prevention campaign and is an expert on reproductive aging.

Before the curtain closes entirely, fertility becomes gradually less reliable in the 10 years leading up to menopause (known as premenopause, or sometimes loosely referred to as perimenopause—the time "around" menopause). RESOLVE: The National Infertility Association aptly describes premenopausal fertility as "decreased, but not entirely absent." But how much a woman's fertility is affected in the transitional period going into menopause is highly individualized.

It's not uncommon for women only in their mid- to late thirties to take fertility drugs because their cycles have already begun to fizzle. Other women conceive through their early and middle forties with ease—including Cherie Blair, the wife of the British prime minister, who had her fourth child at the age of 46 (when she wasn't even trying). There are also unusual cases of women who managed to achieve natural conception even later, such as a California *grandmother* of 13 who made national news in 2002 after giving birth to triplets, which she reportedly conceived naturally at the age of 54.

"If you make a chart of age-related fertility, it would not have a straight line of decline," explains reproductive epidemiologist Shanna H. Swan, Ph.D., research professor in the department of family and community medicine at the University of Missouri–Columbia. It starts out lower since menstrual cycles aren't reliable in early puberty, goes up to its max in late adolescence, and declines slightly throughout the late twenties and early thirties. That decline starts to go down steeply around age 35, says Dr. Swan. The next largest, and sharpest, decline comes around the age of 45 for most women, according to the U.S. Census Bureau, as women are within just about 6 years of the average age of menopause, about 51. To put it into perspective, experts often cite the odds that for women in their forties, the chance of conceiving in any one cycle is about half of what it was in their twenties.

"I counsel women who don't plan to conceive until around age 40 that they are taking the chance of not having fertilizable oocytes (eggs). Chronological age is not the only predictor of fertility, but it must be considered," says Wanda Ronner, M.D., a gynecologist at Pennsylvania Hospital of the University of Pennsylvania Health System in Philadelphia and coauthor of *The Empty Cradle: Infertility in America from Colonial Times to the Present*.

Fortunately, there are other variables, and we can control them a whole lot more than when we might get our first hot flash. "Actions people take long before they may be ready to have children can impact their ability to eventually conceive," the ASRM campaign says.

"In many cases, it's not necessarily age itself that is compromising fertility in older women as much as that by the time women are 35 or over, they have simply had more opportunities to develop conditions that cause infertility," Dr. Metzger explains.

"Just like diseases such as lung cancer or HIV/AIDS, infertility can often be prevented," the ASRM campaign states.

REDUCING YOUR RISKS

In the following pages, the top fertility experts in the world—including the scientists who run the most cutting-edge research labs, the doctors who head the world's leading fertility programs, mind–body visionaries, and preeminent health care practitioners—share their specific insights into what can either compromise or optimize fertility over time. Together, their expert guidelines offer protection for each major facet of fertility: the eggs and sperm themselves, the sexual organs, the hormones, your overall health, and your psyche.

One of the clearest risks to the reproductive organs are sexually transmitted diseases (STDs), which can block a woman's fallopian tubes, toughen up her uterus with scar tissue, or bring on the devastation of cervical cancer. They also contribute to cancer and tubal disorders in men. You will be coached throughout this book to practice prevention of and early intervention for STDs.

The same baby bottle that was portrayed as an hourglass is also pictured in the ASRM campaign as an ashtray, with the message: "If you smoke, this might be your only use for a baby's bottle." The hard-hitting slogan is targeted to both genders, since sperm and egg quality is pro-

WHAT WORKED FOR US

SHE "ADVERTISED" FOR A HUSBAND TO GET A MOVE ON MOTHERHOOD

Because of the rigors of medical school, Mary Jane Minkin, M.D., has a reputation for encouraging the students she mentors at Yale University to wait until they finish their residencies to have children. The obstetrician/gynecologist practiced what she preaches and stayed child-free during her own residency. In fact, her practice was already established for several years when she started thinking more seriously about motherhood.

"I had a great career, lived in a nice town, and stayed on top of my health. I would have been completely ready to start a family at that point, if I had the father picked out. The problem was, I live in a small New England community where I already knew everybody," she says.

Dr. Minkin took out an ad in *New York* magazine, hoping to meet someone who shared her interests. Her exact specifications were met in a mathematician who also runs marathons, plays bridge, listens to classical music, and loves to travel.

As it turns out, Dr. Minkin's mate came along just in the nick of time. The couple conceived their first child when she was 35, but by the time they were trying for child number two, she already had some premenopausal symptoms. She started on medication to normalize her cycles and was pregnant in 2 months, at 37.

Her relatively older pregnancies were problem-free, which she attributes to her long-time commitment to fitness (she swims and runs half-marathons) and to following the nutrition and self-care advice she gives as a *Prevention* magazine columnist. (Think lots of fruits and vegetables, stress management, and appropriate nutritional supplements.)

In her profession, Dr. Minkin is all too aware that pregnancies get riskier over time—which is one reason why she was proactive about starting her family as soon as her ducks were in a row. "If I had met my husband earlier, I probably would have had my kids 5 years earlier," she admits. "But as I tell my patients and students, you can't settle for anyone just to have a kid."

She acknowledges that women may have to bide some time before they are in a good, stable relationship; improve their health status; or become more established professionally. "I firmly believe that you should get pregnant only when you are ready emotionally, financially, and personally," Dr. Minikin says. "If that time doesn't come along until later in your life, I can assure you that if you stay in good health, you have an excellent chance of having a complication-free pregnancy and healthy children, like I did."

foundly threatened by cigarette smoke as well as other substance abuses. In fact, a woman can lose so many eggs by smoking that it can speed up her passage into menopause by 3 years. Experts also emphasize that anyone who wants to conceive should make every effort to avoid second-hand smoke, which contains more than 60 carcinogens that can threaten reproductive health. (For more information about the fertility-robbing effects of smoking, see chapter 4.)

The ubiquitous ASRM baby bottle is also squeezed with measuring tape to relate that "12 percent of all infertility cases are a result of either weighing too much or too little." Weight, fitness, and nutrition play major roles in the maintenance of reproductive hormones. Chapter 5 is devoted to helping you achieve your best fertility weight, while chapter 16 offers a complete hormone-balancing strategy. And because a mighty immune system is necessary to prevent hormone disorders, structural problems, and high-risk pregnancies, plenty of guidelines will be included on a diet and lifestyle that keep the immune system in top form.

While basic good health is the backbone of reproductive health, there are other fertility-protective steps. When going about their day-to-day business, women need to be conscious of the fact that they are carrying precious cargo in their ovaries, experts caution. Certain chromosomal abnormalities responsible for the greater number of birth defects and miscarriages in later-age pregnancies are often simply blamed on "old eggs." But they can actually be the result of cumulative exposure to radiation or mutation-causing chemicals, RESOLVE reports. Chapter 14 offers specific advice on reducing your day-to-day exposure to various forms of radiation, while chapter 9 will teach you to reduce environmental toxins that you probably didn't even realize were there.

"You do not have to give up all of life's little indulgences in order to conceive and carry a healthy baby, but you do have to moderate," states M. Kelly Shanahan, M.D., chair of the obstetrics and gynecology department at Barton Memorial Hospital in South Lake Tahoe, California; director of the Emerald Bay Center for Women's Health in South Lake Tahoe; and author of *Your Over-35 Week-by-Week Pregnancy Guide.*

Rather than overemphasizing your chronological age, this book supports the position that the best marker for how fertile you are and how fertile you will be in the future depends largely on how well you've managed your risk factors over the years. The concept of "preconception care"—which usually refers to health modifications recommended to a couple just as they are trying for a family—has been expanded to include all the years leading up to conception. "With a longer-term focus, you won't get to conception time and have months of work to do, or worse, find out that you (or your partner) developed a fertility problem years ago," explains Dr. Metzger.

HIGH-TECH TO THE RESCUE?

Around the same time that contraception became widely available in the 1960s, so did fertility drugs. Giving eggs an added push to mature and ovulate, these drugs can often restore or improve fertility in a woman whose own hormone regulation system is dysfunctional. In 1981, the first baby was born through in vitro fertilization, the first of the assisted reproductive technologies (ARTs) to introduce sperm and egg outside the body and guide the implantation process. By 1987, these procedures could also be performed with donor eggs, and 10 years later, the use of frozen embryos also became possible (sperm preservation had already been around since the 1970s). Today, scientists are rapidly developing the technology to freeze eggs and pieces of ovaries, advances that should be routinely available in the next 5 years.

Each time one of these new technologies is introduced, a flood of publicity surrounds it, and hopeful couples rush to infertility clinics looking for a miracle. Among those who seek treatment are inevitably healthy and very fertile women in their thirties who panic, prematurely, because they have heard so much about "the infertility problem." "I call these women pre-infertile," says Dr. Ronner. Infertility rates for all ages have actually remained relatively stable over the past 3 decades, but the increasing availability of infertility services has created a misperception of an infertility epidemic, according to the Centers for Disease Control and Prevention. Dr. Ronner counsels her "pre-infertile" patients—who tend to be thirtysomething professional women eager to do everything the right way—that it's normal for them to expect a year of unprotected intercourse before conceiving.

"When it comes to women in their forties and their late thirties, it's reasonable to expect even longer than a year to get pregnant. However, women over 35 are encouraged to be evaluated and possibly go into treatment before a year is up, because our interventions work better when you're younger. So you have to weigh the two," says Steven Sondheimer, M.D., professor of obstetrics and gynecology at the University of Pennsylvania Medical Center in Philadelphia and a spokesperson for the Association of Reproductive Health Professionals.

"In my practice, it's always the goal to see if a woman with fertility problems can conceive on her own by correcting any underlying imbalances in her health and lifestyle. Of course, if a woman is close to menopause, we do this as efficiently as possible," says Dr. Metzger. (For more on Dr. Metzger's holistic approach to fertility problems, see "Fertility Visionaries" on page 12.) Even if a woman has to get high-tech treatment, Dr. Metzger says, if you haven't optimized her immune system and psychological health, you're probably wasting her time and money—which feasibly could be $50,000 worth of treatment not covered by insurance.

In contrast to "pre-infertile" women who jump the gun by seeking high-tech treatment when it's not necessary, "too many women are working under the assumption that they will have no problem getting pregnant once they make the decision to have a child, based on all the advances in infertility treatment," comments Dr. Cullins. An older woman may be devastated to discover that the infertility treatment she expected to fall back on offers very low success rates because of her age. The 16 percent success rate projected for 40-year-old women seeking ARTs drops down to 6 percent by the age of 43 and less than 3 percent after that. Because of poor odds, many clinics exclude women over the age of 43 from services, unless they agree to use another woman's eggs.

It's understandable to want to have something to fall back on—especially for the many women who are acutely aware of that baby-bottle hourglass but can't simply conjure up the right mate, support, or emotional readiness, says Dr. Cullins. But as far as safety nets go, high-tech infertility

FERTILITY VISIONARIES

Deborah Metzger, M.D., Ph.D., and Helena Women's Health

As a reproductive endocrinologist and internationally sought-out gynecologic surgeon, Deborah Metzger, M.D., Ph.D., medical director of Helena Women's Health in San Jose, California, and medical advisor to this book, can easily pull out the big guns for patients with reproductive problems. But rather than jumping into invasive infertility tests, she's more likely to first check for allergies, intestinal bacteria, and high insulin levels. Before she prescribes fertility drugs, she's more likely to prescribe a massage, flaxseed oil, and organic food.

During Dr. Metzger's early years as a reproductive endocrinologist, she found that she could surgically correct a woman's blocked tubes or give her medication that would stabilize her irregular menstrual cycles, but the woman still might not conceive. Just as frustrating was when a woman lost the pregnancy after thinking her problem was "fixed." Dr. Metzger started looking deeper. What she found was that sometimes the simplest and gentlest changes in people's overall well-being help them feel more energetic than they have in years, set them free of chronic pain, and simultaneously give them the capacity to have the children they weren't sure they could.

"In the interest of caring for the whole person and not just the ovaries or the sperm, we have developed an integrated approach to fertility enhancement at Helena Women's Health," Dr. Metzger explains. Drawing on both Western and Eastern medicine, and both high-tech procedures and natural medicine, Dr. Metzger and her staff of nurse-practitioners, nutritionists, mind–body therapists, allergists, and psychotherapists give clients a personalized program to follow for a 3- to 12-month period.

"The most overlooked fertility factor is the health of the immune system," Dr. Metzger says. "Ovulation, implantation, and development of the placenta

treatment is riddled with holes. Costs, medical risks, moral qualms, and advanced age exclude many couples from having ART as an option.

Instead, the best security is knowledge and self-care, our experts say. Knowing your body, trusting your body, and giving it what it needs over

are all dependent on its optimal function." To charge up a patient's immune system, she may need to correct yeast overgrowth, viral diseases, inadequate nutrition, hormonal imbalances, or reactions to food, hormones, or airborne allergens. One way she can help is with immunotherapy—a system of neutralizing allergies faster and more permanently than classic allergy treatment.

Every patient is taught how to eat a low-glycemic diet—not only because sugar disturbs the immune system but because insulin problems are another commonly overlooked fertility factor. Sophisticated tests are offered to assess environmental health as patients learn to avoid chemical toxins and improve their digestion. Patients have a full array of stress-management options to try, including acupuncture, psychotherapy, support groups, and jin shin jyutsu. If clients still need infertility treatment after this, they are in a much better position for it to work, Dr. Metzger explains.

Probably because of its integrative approach, Helena Women's Health has developed a reputation for particularly helping women who have had unsuccessful in vitro fertilization treatments, multiple pelvic surgeries, and other difficult cases. Several hundred women a year come for fertility enhancement.

Contact information: Helena Women's Health is located at 2101 Forest Avenue, Suite 220, San Jose, CA 95128. You can reach them at (408) 999-7900 or via www.helenahealth.com. Out-of-town patients get their initial assessments over the phone by answering a substantial lifestyle survey and going over their complete medical history. Testing and resources are tightly scheduled when patients arrive for a week-long stay. So many women flock in for endometriosis treatment that a local bed-and-breakfast is known as the "Endo Inn."

the years will go a long way in your ability to conceive naturally. Chapters 2 to 14 offer the information you need to do this. And if you haven't discovered this book until after developing fertility problems, chapters 15 to 19 include proven, low-tech solutions from complementary practitioners throughout the world.

CONCEIVE MORE EFFICIENTLY TODAY OR TOMORROW

With knowledge and self-care, it's possible for today's women to be more fertile than their foremothers—despite the trend of delayed childbearing. A prominent British study set out to compare fertility rates from the 1960s through the 1990s, based on the common marker of the time it takes to become pregnant. Much to the researchers' surprise, 80 percent of couples conceived after trying for 6 months in 1991 and 1993, compared to 65 percent of couples between 1961 and 1965. After 1 year, 90 percent of the couples in the 1990s conceived, compared to 79 percent in the 1960s! Women starting families at the end of the 20th century appeared to compensate for their slight biological disadvantages of later-age childbearing with improved nutrition, greater health advantages, and better sexual education (particularly, their knowledge of the menstrual cycle).

"There's no question that people today are healthier in a lot of ways, compared to our mothers' generation. People don't smoke as much, and we've practically eliminated reproductive health threats such as tuberculosis," comments Mary Jane Minkin, M.D., a board-certified obstetrician/gynecologist in New Haven, Connecticut; clinical professor at Yale University Medical School; and advisor to *Prevention* magazine. While we have to work hard to reduce the negative influences of modern life on fertility, there are also a lot of positive things already in place that we simply have to optimize, she says.

Even if you haven't picked up this book until you are currently trying to conceive, you'll be delighted to discover how much more efficiently and healthfully you can conceive with enhanced reproductive know-how. Biologists at the National Institute of Environmental Health Sciences (NIEHS) taught women in different age groups how to plan intercourse precisely for their peak day in their 5- to 6-day "fertile windows." Even the oldest members of the study group (ages 35 to 39) achieved per-cycle conception rates of *up to 30 percent*. This is higher than the probabilities normally cited for even the youngest, healthiest members of the population by esteemed organizations such as the ASRM and the American College of Obstetricians and Gynecology. (Twenty percent of women 30 and under and 5 percent of women 40 and over are expected to conceive from month to month.) "If you know when you are ovulating and make sure to have sex accordingly, you will optimize your chances of getting pregnant at any age," comments Dr. Shanahan.

Because perfectly timed intercourse can tremendously enhance the probability of conception—and conceiving efficiently becomes increasingly important as you get closer to menopause—chapter 12 is devoted to the various methods of ovulation awareness (including the natural family planning method used in the NIEHS study). You'll hear about the latest high-tech gadgets as well as the classic, tried-and-true methods, so you can choose a method that suits your personality and lifestyle. As an added advantage, experts will explain the art of conception-specific sex in chapter 13.

But first, to really get you in tune with your body's cycles, experts will take you through the inner workings of the reproductive system in chapter 2. The better you know what's happening inside, the more empowered you will be to monitor your reproductive health over time and make the most of your fertility when you're ready.

2

The Reproductive System, Decade by Decade

Nature's pure determination to carry on is evident in every species that crawls, slithers, swims, flies, or walks the planet. Retracing the journey of their entire lifetime, Pacific salmon swim thousands of miles upstream to release eggs and sperm near their birthplace. Peacocks cart around a dazzling fan several times their size and weight in order to flag down a desirable mate. Flowers have evolved with ever-more-exquisite varieties of colors and pleasing petal arrangements for the ingenious purpose of luring in butterflies and bumblebees who can transport their DNA-containing pollen to another meadow.

Like any other creature, we humans have intricate systems in place to ensure that our species continues. Whether she's finishing her doctoral dissertation, enduring basic training, or hoping for twins, a woman is functioning as a primal, baby-making factory. Every month, for roughly 3 decades of her life, she matures a crop of egg-containing follicles, selects the best egg to ovulate, and develops a thick, enriched bed inside her uterus to welcome a potential embryo.

For the male of our species, nature has made reproduction "readiness" even simpler. Guys don't even run on cycles—their reproductive systems are constantly "on." They make thousands of new sperm every hour of every day.

Yet despite nature's efforts to guarantee our survival as a species, certain aspects of modern life can go *against* our fertile nature, says Jonathan Tilly, Ph.D., director of the Vincent Center for Reproductive Biology at Massachusetts General Hospital in Boston and associate professor of obstetrics, gynecology, and reproductive biology at Harvard Medical School. He teaches women about egg-zapping factors that include smoking, cancer treatment, working around biohazards like solvents, hanging out in bars, exposure to pesticides, and ingesting the by-products of plastic that might leech into our microwaved food. When he lectures to the public on these topics, Dr. Tilly sees women staring at their abdomens.

"The effects of something that eliminates eggs might not show up for 5 or 15 years. But then you'll use up whatever's left in the pipeline and it won't be replenished," Dr. Tilly explains. "I want women to understand how their bodies function and how important their ovarian reserve is. The earlier they make this connection, the more proactive they can be about their long-term fertility."

THE MIRACULOUS MECHANICS OF THE REPRODUCTIVE SYSTEM

In upcoming chapters, we'll explain how to moderate your habits, lifestyle, and exposure to specific environmental threats in order to protect egg quality and quantity, as well as your man's sperm-making capacity and sperm quality. But since reproduction requires more than just sperm and eggs, we've dedicated this chapter to giving you an overview of the life-giving importance of each sexual organ and fertility hormone, as well as how to take care of the whole amazing system.

Grow, Follicle, Grow

Follicles make up the thin layer of fluid-filled cells that shrink-wrap the eggs nestled in our ovaries. They take responsibility for supplying nutrients and hormones needed by the egg at different stages of development. Throughout a woman's reproductive life, groups of several hundred follicles transition from a dormant state to their first growth spurt. Approximately 20 of the best ones are then "tagged" to begin a more rapid growth spurt by the hormone messenger, the aptly named follicle-stimulating hormone (FSH), which is secreted by the pituitary gland. This signals the start of a woman's new menstrual cycle.

Only one of the follicles will complete the process. That "dominant follicle" is like a queen bee that the hive collectively selects to nurture, while the others are "sacrificed" through selective biology. Estrogen manufactured by the dominant follicle serves as its key messenger. Its first mission: alerting the uterus to start thickening its lining (known as the endometrium) from 0.05 millimeter to, eventually, 20 millimeters.

THE FEMALE REPRODUCTIVE SYSTEM

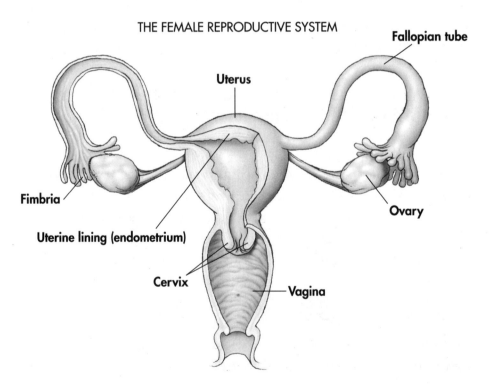

Fallopian tube

Uterus

Fimbria

Ovary

Uterine lining (endometrium)

Cervix

Vagina

By the end of the second week of follicle maturity, there's enough estrogen in the blood to signal the pituitary to blast out a dose of luteinizing hormone (LH). This is around the 14th day of the cycle. A couple hoping to conceive can now get a reading on their ovulation predictor kits, which are designed to pick up that LH surge, and plan a romantic evening. Another hormone exchange occurs when the follicle, having noted the LH surge, sends out progesterone. Progesterone enhances the endometrial growth and maturation that estrogen started.

Simultaneously, LH, estrogen, and progesterone create an alchemy that breaks down the dominant follicle wall, leading to the pivotal moment that an egg emerges. In just 30 minutes after ovulation, the egg passes into the fallopian tube, where it is propelled through a tunnel of waving tentacles known as fimbria. In the first bend of the 10- to 12-centimeter tube, the egg will encounter sperm or will wait for up to 24 hours for a suitor.

Egg, Meet Sperm

Not only has the uterine lining been doing extra housework for its much-anticipated follicular guest, but preparations are being made by the cervix, the connective passage between the vagina and the uterus, for *its* guest. Rather than the sticky, acidic substance it usually makes to discourage intruders (in the form of infections or sperm—or, sometimes, both—arriving nowhere close to ovulation time), the cervix cooks up its equivalent of the welcome mat. "Fertile" cervical mucus is a clear, stretchy stream containing proteins that can keep sperm alive for up to 5 days.

The cervix also rearranges some space for its guest by softening and expanding its walls, which is like opening the front door of the reproductive house. To women who use natural ovulation awareness methods (discussed in chapter 12), these fluid and structural changes are two important signs to look for when deciding whether to have intercourse, depending on whether they want to prevent or promote pregnancy.

In reproductive terms, the object of joining the male and female sexual organs is to merge two fertile bodies of water. Seminal fluid suspending the sperm runs together with the cervical fluid wherever it is deposited along the cervical "riverway" (the higher up, the better its chances). Now, sperm can swim upstream into the "lake" of the uterus and zip up through the narrow tributary of the fallopian tube.

Only the most vigorous, healthy sperm can lash their tails all the way through this network—which is why around 250 million to 400 million of them are deposited in a typical ejaculation (that's for a healthy sperm count of 30 million to 60 million per milliliter of seminal fluid). Before an hour has passed, most of them will poop out while still in the uterus. Others have poor navigational skills and swim up the wrong tube, even though an egg sends chemical radar through the cervical fluid. If one of the 200 or so robust sperm that make it to the egg's lair actually penetrates the egg, a chemical reaction occurs that prevents the others from gaining entrance.

Swapping Genes

The sperm needs to plunge its way through three layers of egg, including a jellylike outer layer, a tough second layer, and, finally, the inner coating, where an electrical charge of sorts exists. The egg, which started expelling half its set of 46 chromosomes at ovulation in preparation for this moment, finishes this process. The sperm head falls apart, presenting its perfect match of 23 chromosomes. The two sets can now "mingle and match"—including the egg's X chromosome and the sperm's X (female) or Y (male) chromosome that will determine their offspring's gender.

The fertilized pre-embryo has already started dividing cells as it leaves its love nest for a 3-day trip through the more narrow end of the fallopian tube. Beating, hairlike cilia, which line the tube, pulse their cargo in the direction of the uterus, while it is sustained by glucose, mucus, and other nourishing fluids from secretory cells in the tubal lining.

The egg sends word that it has been fertilized to its old nest site, the follicle, now known as the corpus luteum. (In a similar process, the mother-to-be may alert her own family about a new member in a few weeks!) After getting the message (in the form of human chorionic gonadotropin, or hCG), the follicle sends forth more progesterone than ever to promote the implantation process. The uterine lining grows another 2 millimeters and secretes "welcoming" fluids.

After 3 days through the tubes and 72 hours of floating around the uterus, the fertilized egg (now called a zygote) sinks itself into the pillowy endometrial lining, ideally in the most secure upper back portion of the uterus. It is about the size of the period at the end of this sentence and has divided into about 107 to 256 cells. The corpus luteum will continue to secrete high levels of estrogen and progesterone, which allows sufficient blood and nutrients to reach the developing embryo. This is particularly crucial before week 10, until the placenta has developed enough to take over some of this role.

Endometrial cells also produce hormones to support the fledgling pregnancy. Prolactin helps develop the placenta (and will eventually stimulate breast milk). Relaxin prevents the uterus from contracting as it would to expel the endometrial lining in the form of monthly menstruation, which occurs when the egg goes unfertilized.

Soon the fetus will be making its own hormone, called human chorionic somatomammotropin, which takes energy stores from the mother for its own use. The early embryo also produces chemicals that establish itself to the mother's immune system as a "friendly foreigner" that's planning on sticking around for another 9 months or so.

WHERE HAVE ALL MY EGGS GONE?

Those who can remember seeing Peter, Paul, and Mary singing the lyrics "where have all the flowers gone" at a flower child festival are most likely, by now, singing their own tune about pining for eggs instead of flowers and soldiers. Even if they haven't hit menopause yet, forty- and fiftysomething women from the baby boomer generation are losing eggs faster than flowers in an early frost.

To put it bluntly, a woman's reproductive system ages more quickly than the rest of her body. By menopause, a woman's bones, uterus, and mucous membranes have to cope with 90 percent less estrogen than they are accustomed to. When it comes to your eggs, your supply started to dwindle before you were even born.

As Dr. Tilly explains, we had approximately seven million eggs as 20-week-old fetuses—and this number went down to six million by our birth. By the time we reached puberty and were able to actually use the eggs, we were left with somewhere around 300,000 to spread out over our reproductive lifetimes. If you do the math and figure that we need only 300 to 400 eggs for all the ovulation we are likely to do between puberty and menopause, then those are pretty good odds. Not all eggs, however, are ovulation-worthy.

"It's the same reason why men ejaculate millions of sperm in order to get a few superior ones that can make it to the eggs—many of them are flawed. Similarly, the female body appears to have imperfect eggs to begin with," says Dr. Tilly. The biological process called apoptosis helps eliminate less-than-desirable eggs. If the apoptosis gene is activated, a cell self-destructs, he explains. Throughout our body, damaged, unwanted, or troublemaking cells are deleted through this process. "In the last 10 years, we've come to understand that apoptosis is how the body fights off cancer," Dr. Tilly notes. It also protects us from autoimmune disease by deleting cells that would prey on our own body, he says.

Bax, the gene that orders apoptosis in unwanted cells, seems very responsible—until you realize that it could nearly deplete a woman's follicle reserve by the time she reaches middle age. In fact, the apoptosis process in our ovaries speeds up as we get closer to menopause. That's why at 40, a woman's body may have only five follicles or fewer to choose from when selecting the dominant follicle in a given cycle, compared to a younger woman who might have as many as 50 potential contenders.

Amazingly, Dr. Tilly and his Harvard research partners are learning how to tone down Bax. They have retarded follicular apoptosis so successfully that mice aged equivalent to 80-year-old women had eggs that fertilized and developed into embryos. But don't count on a pill or procedure to preserve your eggs before your first hot flash—it's going to be tricky to tell Bax to spare eggs but zap cancer and other troublesome cells, he says.

Besides, even if we can alter egg quantity, there's no therapy that can change the age-related decline in egg *quality*.

Questionable Chromosomes

"Just like a chef reaches for the most pleasing ingredients from his pantry first, it appears that your reproductive system has a way of using more of its prime egg stock earliest in life," says Michael Soules, M.D., professor of obstetrics and gynecology at the University of Washington in Seattle and an expert on reproductive aging. It's not that all of the eggs left in later years are the equivalent of that dusty box of macaroni and cheese at the back of the pantry shelf. But a larger proportion of eggs with genetic defects are left over in our "back stock" as we get older, he explains.

Fortunately, apoptosis zaps many of the irregulars as they come out of dormancy, so that the egg you do ovulate is more likely to come from the "top shelf." If genetically flawed eggs do make it to ovulation, a second line of quality control may occur when the sperm fails to fertilize the egg or the chromosomes fail to divide, explains reproductive endocrinologist and gynecologic surgeon Deborah Metzger, M.D., Ph.D., medical director of Helena Women's Health in San Jose, California, and medical advisor to this book. The egg may have been fine to begin with, but since older chromosomes are "stickier" (after all, they've been together for so many years), they might have trouble organizing the genetic material to form an embryo, she points out.

If chromosomally abnormal embryos do manage to form, they are categorized as aneuploid (the wrong number of chromosomes), polyploid (multiple copies of the same chromosomes), or mosaic (different cells with different chromosomal makeups). Scientists aren't sure how often these embryos form only to self-destruct shortly afterward, because it happens before a woman has detectable signs of pregnancy.

Our third level of quality control is the body's instinct to abort a flawed embryo after it implants in the uterus. Scientists suspect that half of all miscarriages occur when chromosomally abnormal embryos fail to grow or develop normally. In women up to age 35, about 10 percent of pregnancies are known to end in miscarriage. But largely due to more chromosomal issues, this number nearly doubles for women between 35 and 39 and doubles again after 5 more years.

Despite these surveillance mechanisms, women of all ages still bring chromosomally abnormal children to term. The most well-known disorder is Down syndrome, in which children are born with an extra chromosome 21. Statistically, at the age of 25, 1 in 1,250 women give birth to a baby with Down syndrome. The odds increase to 1 in 400 by age 35, 1 in 100 at age 40, and 1 in 30 by age 45. The age-related rise is similar for other genetic disorders.

On the brighter side, if prenatal testing rules out chromosomal defects, an older woman in good health can have confidence that her baby probably is at no greater risk of birth defects than if she were in her twenties, according to the March of Dimes. About 95 percent of women who undergo prenatal testing receive the reassuring news that their babies do not have a chromosomal disorder.

Despite all this talk about things that can go haywire, don't get the idea that because he or she was spawned from your older egg, your child will necessarily have physical or mental disadvantages growing up, Dr. Soules clarifies. "Either there is a genetic anomaly or there is not. There aren't subtle gene defects that subtly compromise the offspring born to older parents," he assures.

Erratic Hormones

One of the first signs that our reproductive system is going south is when the hormonal relay system described earlier develops miscommunications.

Remember that FSH is secreted by the pituitary gland to induce egg maturation within the ovary. Think of older follicles as a little hard of hearing, just like their middle-aged owners who grew up listening to The Rolling Stones. The pituitary gland may have to send down more FSH—which is like yelling at the follicle to perform. This coping strategy of elevated FSH may work for a while, nudging some of the last few thousand follicles to mature.

;h, follicles don't respond at all, or when they do, they
for ovulation. Some follicles fail to send enough es-
ie ahead to prepare the uterine lining for the egg's
. The feedback system may temporarily regain con-
et back on schedule for a few more months—before
se are all indications of impending menopause.
chapter 1, women enter menopause at different
within each age group fertility varies tremendously.
fertility decline intensifies as we get closer to our
knowing how far we are from menopause sheds
)ductive age and helps us make informed child-

..y. Although the average age for menopause is 50,
omen whose mothers entered menopause earlier or later than this have
about a 50 percent chance of mirroring their mothers' patterns. There are
many other factors that could influence the age a woman enters
menopause, but none have such a clear influence as her mother's age, says
Dr. Metzger. Theoretically, a woman could have "saved" some eggs for her
later years if she entered puberty later than usual, or during the times she
didn't ovulate because of pregnancy, breastfeeding, or hormonal contraceptives.

We also know that some lifestyle factors tend to be hard on the ovaries,
such as smoking, alcoholism, obesity, and exposure to toxins (everything
from pollution to pesticides, as you will read in chapter 9). "It's tempting
to try to come up with some kind of a formula where you add a few years
for this and subtract a few years for that. But besides one's mother's age,
we don't know the relative weight of any other factors enough to develop
an accurate prediction," explains Dr. Metzger. Making matters more complicated is that reproductive aging also differs among races, cultures, geo-
graphic regions, and socioeconomic statuses.

Since hormone activity offers some important clues, doctors will make
rough estimates of your age-related reproductive capacity based on your
levels of FSH, estrogen, and other reproductive hormones. But the way

these levels fluctuate doesn't make them reliable enough to draw any absolute conclusions. "Every fertility doctor has seen a woman with a high perimenopausal FSH level who went on to conceive naturally," says Mary Jane Minkin, M.D., a board-certified obstetrician/gynecologist in New Haven, Connecticut; clinical professor at Yale University Medical School; and advisor to *Prevention* magazine.

YOUR "REAL" REPRODUCTIVE AGE

Up until 2001, there were no clinical guidelines to characterize our reproductive life span. Finally, representatives from esteemed organizations, including the American Society for Reproductive Medicine (ASRM), the National Institutes of Health, and the North American Menopause Society, pooled their knowledge and developed the STRAW system. STRAW stands for the Stages of Reproductive Aging Workshop in which it was developed, under the direction of Dr. Soules.

The beauty of STRAW is that you can get a sense of what stage you are in based on your menstrual patterns, symptoms, and the *overall characteristics* of a stage, rather than just a certain hormone range or chronological age. Looking at the whole picture makes it clearer that reproductive capacity is unique for each individual, explains Dr. Soules. After all, there are a great number of variables in each woman's genetic makeup, health, and lifestyle habits that carry her more quickly or slowly from one reproductive stage to another.

Even the stages designated by STRAW aren't set in stone. "While most women will progress from one stage to the next, some will seesaw between stages or skip a stage altogether," says Dr. Soules. It's also important to keep in mind that although normal menopause occurs between 42 and 58, the age ranges in STRAW are based on the average age of 50 (so you can feasibly be up to 8 years ahead of or behind the curve).

Note that while the stages are based on the STRAW model, our experts not affiliated with STRAW have also commented on fertility issues to be aware of at each stage.

Early Reproductive Stage

Approximate age: Puberty to age 20

Hormone levels: Your FSH and estrogen are within normal range (although you probably have no reason to have them tested).

Characteristics: Following your first period, your menstrual cycles may take several years to fall into the 28- to 31-day pattern that you can expect for the majority of your reproductive years. Your hormone feedback system may not be strong enough to always induce ovulation, which is one reason why sexually active women in this stage are slightly less fertile than their more mature sisters.

Fertility issues: "Women in this generation are the only group whose smoking rates are on the rise. That's very bad news, because you may be killing off without any trace a substantial number of eggs that you'll wish you had 15 years down the line, especially if you expect to delay childbearing," says Dr. Tilly.

Stage-specific advice: Single, teen mothers are the most economically disadvantaged group in the nation. "Planning childbearing with your career in mind and waiting for a supportive partner are perfectly legitimate reasons to delay childbearing," says American culture scholar Margaret Marsh, Ph.D., professor of history and dean of the faculty of arts and sciences at Rutgers University in Camden, New Jersey, and coauthor of *The Empty Cradle: Infertility in America from Colonial Times to the Present.*

Middle Reproductive Stage

Approximate age: 20 to 38

Hormone levels: Your FSH and estrogen are within normal range (you might want to get a baseline test at around age 35).

Characteristics: Your menstrual cycles should be regular throughout this stage. One percent of the female population, however, experiences menopause before the age of 40, where FSH levels prematurely increase and menstrual cycles stop (see the discussion of premature ovarian failure later in this chapter).

Fertility issues: This is the longest of all the stages. It's actually broken into three segments. The first 7 years are your *peak fertility time;* the next third marks your first slight fertility decline, followed by the beginning of your second fertility decline, around age 35. (The sharpest statistical drop in fertility, however, occurs at the age of 45, according to the U.S. Census Bureau.)

Stage-specific advice: Sexually transmitted diseases (STDs) are highest among women in their twenties, and they're the leading cause of infertility for this generation. "The greatest long-term fertility advice we doctors can give is to avoid STDs by practicing safe sex," says Wanda Ronner, M.D., a gynecologist at Pennsylvania Hospital of the University of Pennsylvania Health System in Philadelphia and coauthor with Dr. Marsh of *The Empty Cradle: Infertility in America from Colonial Times to the Present.*

Late Reproductive Stage

Approximate age: 38 to 42

Hormone levels: Your FSH levels may have jumped from around 5 mIU/mL to closer to 15 or 20. If a test indicates that your FSH levels are normal and you're already 40, have the test taken a second time, since levels in this stage tend to fluctuate from month to month.

Characteristics: Although your FSH levels may have increased, you probably still ovulate and menstruate on your usual 28- to 31-day schedule. But since your follicles are getting less responsive to FSH, they may produce less estrogen. As the body's estrogen receptors take note, you may become more sensitive to extreme temperatures or even experience hot flashes. Since lower estrogen levels affect the elasticity and acidity of the vagina, you may need a lubricant during sex or develop more yeast and bladder infections than you did in younger years. Even if you didn't get PMS in the past, you're now more likely to experience mood swings and discomfort around the time of your period.

Fertility issues: Your natural increase in FSH may be so stimulating to the ovary that it brings more than one egg to maturity. That's why if you were to get pregnant in your late thirties, you're more likely to have multiple births! (This probability drops off in your forties, unless you use fertility drugs, which also promote multiple births.) And since birth defects increase in women over 35, you are advised to consider genetic counseling before conceiving.

Stage-specific advice: "The first sign of elevated FSH is a call to accelerate your childbearing plans, particularly if you wish to conceive without medical intervention in the future," says Dr. Metzger. To maintain your ovulation consistency, you may want to consider natural supplements such as vitex (described in chapter 16) or, if you are currently trying to conceive, a prescription for clomiphene citrate (Clomid).

Early Perimenopausal Stage

Approximate age: 42 to 46

Hormone levels: Your FSH may have doubled from the last stage, up to around 30 mIU/mL. Estrogen could be declining (under 80 pg/mL) due to lower follicle quantity and quality, or it may be temporarily elevated (above 100 pg/mL) in an attempt to modulate high FSH.

Characteristics: As you get deeper into the menopausal transition, not only is the follicle releasing less estrogen, it's also skimping on progesterone, which normally soars in the second half of your cycle. With only moderate amounts of estrogen stimulating the uterus, and no progesterone, there's less uterine lining to shed, and you do so earlier in your cycle. Consequently, your cycles may shorten to 24 to 27 days instead of 28 to 31, and your periods might be heavier or lighter than they used to be.

Fertility issues: Pregnancy and labor may require more medical attention for women over 40. You are almost twice as likely to have a cesarean birth as younger women, have a 7 percent chance of developing gestational diabetes (compared to 1.7 percent for a woman in her twenties), and are more likely to experience high blood pressure in pregnancy (even if you didn't have it already). Hopefully, you've kept up with a fitness program and optimized your nutrition as part of your preconception care plan—which can help you beat the odds for high-risk pregnancies, says Dr. Minkin.

Stage-specific advice: Whether or not you have opted to use medical intervention like fertility drugs or in vitro fertilization (IVF) to increase your chances of conception, make sure you ask your doctor about taking progesterone to help the uterine lining build up enough for a fertilized egg to implant and stick, urges Dr. Metzger.

Late Perimenopausal Stage

Approximate age: 46 to 50

Hormone levels: Your FSH levels continue to climb, typically as high as 50 mIU/mL.

Characteristics: Even if your very high FSH successfully stimulates a follicle to mature, that follicle can be "deaf" to the next signal down the line, which is LH and its cohort hormones telling it to release the egg. Expect ovulation to be hit or miss—this stage is characterized by two or more skipped menstrual cycles. And then, just when you thought you could stop clipping tampon coupons, your period might come back. It may be a "phantom period" where you don't ovulate but still have some endometrium to shed, or you may resume your old ovulation pattern for a few more months or years. The less frequently you ovulate, the less estrogen you produce—which often means more noticeable perimenopause symptoms.

Fertility issues: Mentally prepare yourself for pregnancy loss, since *half* of pregnancies to women over 45 end in miscarriage. "And since childbirth is more aerobic than a half marathon, it's essential that you are physically 'trained' before conceiving. At the least, try to walk 3 miles every other day," says Dr. Minkin.

Stage-specific advice: "When considering if you have what it takes to *raise* the child to adulthood, apply the hoop-shooting rule: Ask yourself if you will be energetic and fit enough to shoot hoops with your child on their 13th birthday," Dr. Minkin advises.

Menopause and Postmenopausal Stage

Approximate age: 50+

Hormone levels: Your FSH levels will reach their peak, between about 50 and 70 mIU/mL, where they will stay. Your ovaries significantly decrease their production of estrogen, although the adrenal glands continue to produce small amounts.

Characteristics: Once you haven't had a period for an entire year, you're officially in menopause. You can now be almost certain of not flip-flopping back into a surprise ovulatory cycle. Of interest, you may still have a few hundred or even a few thousand eggs in your follicles, but the last few hundred generally don't develop.

Fertility issues: Your last option for getting pregnant now may be the high-tech medical intervention of using a donor egg with an IVF treatment—that is, if you have the financial capability and your doctors think you're likely to respond. When over-40 women undergo IVF with younger women's eggs, they actually have very similar conception rates as younger women. In order to truly "level the playing field," though, older women may need to have more embryos transferred than younger women would and take progesterone along with standard fertility drugs. You may also want to flip to chapter 19 to learn more about adoption.

Stage-specific advice: The ASRM advises women to have counseling to understand the full legal, ethical, psychological, and social issues involved with using donor eggs or sperm. In fact, RESOLVE: The National Infertility Association recommends that both the couple receiving the egg and the donor of the egg work with a lawyer.

READING YOUR GYNECOLOGICAL VITAL SIGNS

"Think of your menstrual cycle as a vital sign, and any abnormalities you notice in it should be treated with the same vigor as other abnormal vital signs, like pulse," stresses Lawrence Nelson, M.D., a gynecological endocrinology researcher in the women's health branch of the National Institutes of Health.

In most cases, we will have symptoms and signs that something is wrong in enough time to correct it, without organ-robbing surgery or infertility becoming our fate, says Dr. Metzger. Routine screenings during your annual exam will catch a lot, so be sure to see your ob/gyn every year, she stresses. "A yearly Pap test is your best bet for early diagnosis of cervical cancer. Your doctor can also answer your general health questions and spot early warning signs for conditions such as uterine fibroids, thyroid disease, polycystic ovarian syndrome, and breast cancer."

If anything unusual occurs before your next exam, however, it's essential to report it to your doctor. Pelvic inflammatory disease is a prime example of the importance of early intervention. What starts out as minor symptoms of genital itching, abnormal discharge, mild discomfort, and irritation can be treated and cured in the first few days with a simple antibiotic prescription. But left untreated for a few more days, and that infection is like a wildfire that sweeps up your reproductive tract, inflaming and permanently scarring the reproductive organs.

In order to prevent future problems—or catch them before they progress to the point of infertility—the following guide will help you to take a proactive approach to gynecological issues that could arise throughout your life.

Dysfunctional uterine bleeding (DUB)/hyperplasia. Menstrual bleeding is considered excessive if you soak more than one pad or tampon every 2 hours or bleed for more than 7 days. Sometimes this happens if the hormone changes of perimenopause cause the uterine lining to build up during missed cycles. You could also have hyperplasia, a hormone-mediated thickening of the uterine lining. Since hyperplasia occasionally leads to cancer, don't delay getting a biopsy to rule out malignancy, in addition to a full medical exam to rule out hemophilia and other bleeding disorders and other suspicious causes. DUB is also often associated with polycystic ovary syndrome (PCOS), otherwise known as Stein–Leventhal disease, which is discussed later in this chapter. Although bleeding can be so disruptive that drastic steps are tempting, remember that ablation and hysterectomy render you sterile (see "Before You Go under the Knife" on page 34 for other options).

Preventive steps: Hyperplasia appears to be aggravated by estrogen, so be proactive by embracing the hormone-balancing dietary and detoxification recommendations discussed in chapter 16. You'll also want to follow the strategies described in chapter 9 for avoiding endocrine-disrupting chemicals.

Endometriosis. This fertility hazard leaves a menacing calling card: severe menstrual cramping that may also be accompanied by intense bloating, vomiting, and heavier-than-normal bleeding during your period. You may also be struck with pain during urination, elimination, or intercourse. Other symptoms include backache, chronic fatigue, gastrointestinal upset, and urinary trouble (frequent voiding, or difficulty producing a stream of urine). Endometriosis is characterized by tissue that breaks off from the uterine lining and implants in other parts of the body. Not only does this cause uncomfortable inflammation, but the scar tissue building up on your organs makes endometriosis a leading fertility problem.

Preventive steps: Since endometriosis is aggravated by estrogen, hormone-balancing lifestyle interventions are in order, including the dietary and detoxification recommendations in chapter 16 and the steps to avoid endocrine-disrupting chemicals explained in chapter 9. Also, the Physicians' Committee on Responsible Medicine (PCRM) reports that women who work out at least 2 hours a week have half the risk of endometriosis as nonexercisers. PCRM also reports that high caffeine consumption is linked to the disease.

Fibroids. Otherwise known as leiomyoma, these smooth-muscle growths in or around the uterus may cause pelvic pain or heavy menstrual bleeding. They may also cause pain during intercourse, back or leg aches, and urinary trouble (frequent voiding, urinary tract infections). Otherwise, they don't always have symptoms, but your gynecologist may feel them during your annual exam. Two to three out of 10 women have these growths, which may cause no fertility problems at all (even during pregnancy) or may meddle with pregnancy by causing infertility, miscarriage, premature birth, or labor and delivery problems. (Read more in chapter 17.) Fibroids account for one-third of all hysterectomies performed in the United States and two-thirds of the hysterectomies of African-American women—but this number wouldn't be nearly so high if early intervention were done, says Dr. Metzger.

(continued on page 37)

BEFORE YOU GO UNDER THE KNIFE

More than half a million hysterectomies a year are performed in the United States, half of them in women still in their reproductive years. Yet the Centers for Disease Control and Prevention reports studies suggesting that 15 percent of hysterectomies may be unnecessary—and other women's health advocates claim that more than 75 percent could be avoided.

"Unless you have cancer, or you are bleeding to death, you don't have to have the organs of your reproductive system removed," says Mary Jane Minkin, M.D., an obstetrician/gynecologist in New Haven, Connecticut; clinical professor at Yale University Medical School; and advisor to *Prevention* magazine. If you're not 100 percent certain that you are finished childbearing, you'll be glad to know that there are alternatives.

According to reproductive endocrinologist and gynecologic surgeon Deborah Metzger, M.D., Ph.D., medical director of Helena Women's Health in San Jose, California, and medical advisor to this book, women aren't always presented their full spectrum of options, because some doctors push only the procedures that they've had training to perform themselves. That's why the Centers for Disease Control and Prevention advises that you get a second opinion any time a doctor wants to remove your organs.

"Consult with infertility specialists, who are more likely to perform sophisticated, organ-sparing procedures like the myomectomy," Dr. Metzger advises. "Ask your doctor to explain every procedure that's available to treat your problem. If surgery is recommended, make sure you've been given a very good reason," she says. Of course, hysterectomy can greatly improve the quality of life for women with intensely disruptive symptoms, so it should be included among your options.

HYSTERECTOMY ALTERNATIVE

Wait and watch: This legitimate medical approach means that you will undergo regular monitoring to see if your condition becomes more acute before opting for any medication or surgical intervention.

Pro: Hormone-mediated conditions such as endometriosis, fibroids, hyperplasia, cysts, and polyps often disappear on their own, sparing you the costs and risks of surgery or medication.

Con: Certain types of hyperplasia can lead to cancer, so the monitoring you get must be vigilant. Also, by not taking aggressive action on fibroids while they are small, more invasive, higher-risk options may be needed to treat larger growths, Dr. Metzger points out.

Diet and lifestyle management: Practitioners of complementary and Eastern medicine can offer nutrition, herbs, bodywork, mind–body techniques, and gentle symptom-solvers. Acupuncture is particularly promising.

Pro: Unlike many surgical and pharmaceutical options that provide only temporary relief, these methods may permanently correct your problem. By supporting the immune system, you're optimizing overall wellness and your chances to fully heal.

Con: Not likely to produce the instant results you'd get with surgery or pharmaceutical options.

Birth control pills: The Pill is the leading, first line of treatment for shrinking endometrial adhesions and cysts, controlling hyperplasia, and managing PCOS.

Pro: Very reliable birth control for mutually monogamous relationships.

Con: If you stop the Pill and want to conceive, it may take several months for ovulation to resume. Also, birth control pills are associated with a slightly increased risk for cervical cancer.

Gonadotropin-releasing hormone (GnRH) agonist drugs: These may shrink fibroids and relieve endometriosis by decreasing estrogen to menopausal levels.

Pro: May also reduce complications of surgery, if needed.

Con: Can be used only temporarily (for less than 6 months) because they will bring on menopausal symptoms and the side effects of estrogen deprivation.

The levonorgestrel-releasing intrauterine device (IUD) (Mirena): The progesterone in this contraceptive device does wonders for managing heavy bleeding conditions and curbing endometriosis.

Pro: It has proven results—when researchers in Finland asked 56 women with excessive bleeding to try it for 6 months, two-thirds felt better enough to cancel their hysterectomies. Also, extremely reliable (over 99 percent) contraceptive protection and reverses quickly after removal.

Con: Although newer IUDs don't carry the risk of the Dalkon Shield, all IUDs do pose a very slight risk of perforating your internal organs and breeding infection.

(continued)

BEFORE YOU GO UNDER THE KNIFE (cont.)

Myomectomy: A fibroid is cauterized with a laser or electrical needle, or surgically removed, leaving the uterus intact. Depending on the severity of your condition, the procedure will be either minimally invasive when done with a laproscope (a small surgical microscope), or a more complicated "open surgery."

Pro: Literature shows that myomectomy enhances fertility in women who have trouble conceiving.

Con: Cesarean delivery is more common after a myomectomy. Scar tissue (adhesions) results 80 percent of the time, but fertility data argue that the benefits still outweigh the risks.

Uterine embolization: To control dysfunctional bleeding or fibroids, the blood supply to vessels in the uterus is cut off by bombarding them with dissolvable microscopic plastic particles.

Pro: Since it doesn't produce scarring like other surgical procedures, some experts think it's an excellent option for women of childbearing age.

Con: Because the procedure is relatively new, we don't know the long-term effects, including those on fertility. Plus, recovery from the procedure often involves 4 to 5 days of excruciating pain.

Endometrial ablation: The inner lining of the uterus (endometrium) and the layer below it are frozen or stripped away.

Pro: It's a relatively minor procedure since it can be done vaginally.

Con: Definitely not an option for women who want to carry a pregnancy.

Nonradical hysterectomy: The problematic organ (cervix, ovary, fallopian tube, or uterus) is removed, but the others are left alone.

Pro: Donor egg or surrogacy can still make pregnancy a possibility for women losing only the ovaries or uterus, and natural conception may still be possible for those with one out of two ovaries or tubes intact.

Con: The remaining organs are put at risk for damage or infection from the procedure. Also, hysterectomy does not always relieve chronic pelvic pain after all.

Preventive steps: Like endometriosis, fibroids appear to be aggravated by hormones, which means that the same hormone-balancing diet and lifestyle changes mentioned for endometriosis are also appropriate for fibroids. Also, a large Italian study found that women who ate more beef, ham, and other red meat were the most likely to have fibroids, while those who ate more seafood, vegetables, and fruit were more likely to be fibroid-free.

Polycystic ovary syndrome (PCOS). Elevated insulin, excessive testosterone, and increased estrogen are among the hormone imbalances that produce the classic symptoms of PCOS: erratic or nonexistent periods, acne, difficulty losing weight, and masculine traits (hair growth on the face or chest, balding scalp). Other symptoms include a discharge from the nipples, mood swings, and a lightheaded feeling after large meals. You are particularly predisposed to PCOS if your family history includes diabetes, PCOS, or another insulin-sensitive condition. Unmanaged, PCOS carries a higher risk for uterine cancer, heart disease, diabetes, and infertility—so by all means, be evaluated and treated by an endocrinologist well experienced with the syndrome if you're experiencing any of the symptoms mentioned above.

Preventive steps: First and foremost, follow a low-glycemic diet, as described in chapter 3. Second, if you are overweight (half of women diagnosed with PCOS are), be aggressive about daily exercise and smaller meals, which will help your cells respond better to insulin. Third, consider taking birth control pills to keep your menstrual cycles and hormones in sync.

Ovarian cysts. If these fluid-filled sacs grow on the ovaries, they may cause abdominal pressure or bloating. Ninety-eight percent of all cysts resolve on their own within 2 months. Yet while the cysts themselves might not cause infertility, they can be a red flag for other fertility-related problems. Most likely, a woman who forms cysts needs to address hormone problems such as elevated insulin or androgen levels, says Dr. Metzger. It's also important for her doctor to rule out endometriosis and ovarian cancer (fortunately, cysts are almost always benign). Once cysts grow to more than 2 inches, surgery is usually recommended, she adds.

Preventive steps: Birth control pills can prevent cysts. And since cysts may be hormone-mediated, hormone-regulating lifestyle measures are also in order, particularly the low-glycemic diet described in chapter 3.

Premature ovarian failure. Even if you are "too young" for menopause, see your doctor promptly if you start to skip menstrual cycles or they become unpredictable, or you experience classic perimenopause symptoms such as hot flashes, vaginal dryness, and sleep disruption. Women in their teens, twenties, and thirties can experience premature ovarian failure, otherwise known as early menopause. Make sure your doctor gives you a hormone screening (for FSH, estradiol, and, if possible, inhibin B) and doesn't just chalk your symptoms up to stress, advises Dr. Nelson.

"If the condition is diagnosed early enough, an infertility specialist can possibly help you conceive before your ovaries quit completely," notes Dr. Metzger. Even if doctors say there is nothing they can do, 10 percent of women with premature ovarian failure have spontaneous remission (though you shouldn't count on this), and clomiphene citrate (Clomid) may encourage some of the last eggs to develop.

Preventive steps: Know your family history. If early menopause or autoimmune illness runs in your family, you are predisposed to premature ovarian failure and may want to plan to start a family as early as you're possibly ready. You might also want to consider banking your eggs or pieces of your ovaries for future use. In any case, take heed of lifestyle factors that deplete eggs prematurely.

Pelvic inflammatory disease (PID) and STDs. See your doctor promptly (and bring your partner for treatment, too) about any genital itching, genital irritation, back pain that radiates down your legs, abdominal discomfort, or odoriferous discharge. If an infection develops into PID, abdominal discomfort can become so severe you can't walk. As PID spreads to your bloodstream, you'll get classic flulike symptoms, including fever, chills, and joint aches. At that point, rush to the ER. Not only does advanced PID ravage your reproductive organs, it can become life-threatening. You may need intravenous antibiotics and surgery to drain abscesses.

Preventive steps: First and foremost, the best prevention is using condoms during all sexual contact not meant for conception, since PID is usually triggered by STDs. Second, anyone with a history of PID shouldn't use an intrauterine device (IUD) for birth control. (If any infection remains, the device can be like a coral reef for infection to build on and spread.) Third, don't douche; it can push infection deeper into your reproductive organs.

Uterine prolapse. The uterus may tilt away or drop from its position on the wall of the pelvis when the ligaments that hold it in place become weak. One of the first signs is leaking urine, accompanied by a feeling of abdominal pressure. Try to get a diagnosis before the uterus can be seen or felt through the vagina—at that point you need surgery to tighten the ligaments. In fact, 16 percent of hysterectomies are performed because of uterine prolapse.

Preventive steps: Keep the pelvic muscles strong by doing Kegel exercises regularly: Contract the floor of your pelvis as if you were trying to stop the flow of urine, and hold for several seconds. Repeat 10 times in a row, several times a day.

THE AGING MALE REPRODUCTIVE SYSTEM

It is not uncommon for men to become fathers in their seventies and beyond. U.S. Senator Strom Thurmond fathered a child in his eighties!

It's not that sperm quality and quantity don't decrease with age—they do. In fact, researchers at the National Institute of Environmental Health conducted a study that indicates that male fertility starts to decline as early as the late thirties (which is in line with smaller U.S. studies). On the other hand, the predominant research indicates that whatever age-related declines men do experience, they aren't enough to significantly alter overall pregnancy rates.

University of Southern California researchers observed 414 couples who were using eggs from younger donors during an IVF procedure, which ruled out the impact of the female partner's age. They found that the oldest

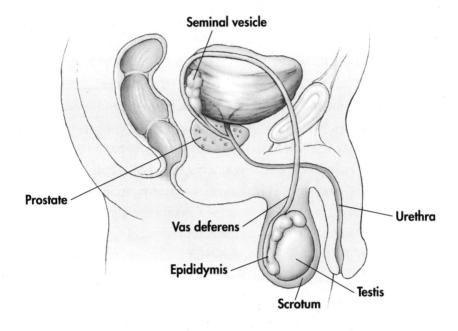

Seminal vesicle

Prostate

Vas deferens

Epididymis

Scrotum

Urethra

Testis

THE MALE REPRODUCTIVE SYSTEM

Each of the illustrated organs plays a vital role in male reproduction.

Testicles. The testicles are essentially the sperm-generating factory, where sperm are created and spend their first 48 days of life. Sertoli cells nourish the sperm during early development, while the Leydig cells produce the testosterone necessary for the sperm to mature.

Scrotum. This sac surrounding the testicles plays the important role of maintaining the proper temperature for the heat- and cold-sensitive sperm-generating factory.

Epididymis. After their first 48 days in the testicles, sperm float into this long coil duct, where they are bathed in nutrients as they mature for 14 more days. Mature sperm will then swim through this duct's 6 meters of tubing, toward the vas deferens.

Vas deferens. This duct connects the sperm from their "nesting site" to their "waiting site." It is the area surgically closed off when a man has a vasectomy.

Seminal vesicles. These pouches store the mature sperm for up to 14 days until they are ready for ejaculation. They also provide the sperm with 80 percent of the seminal fluid they will leave the body with.

Prostate. The prostate gland contributes the additional 20 percent of seminal fluid that mixes with the sperm to form ejaculate.

Urethra. At the time of orgasm, the pelvic muscles, prostate, and lining of the vas deferens contract, propelling semen down this narrow opening through the penis.

men in the group (ages 51 to 64) had the same results as their younger male peers. A comparable Spanish study found that pregnancy rates were similar for the male partner whether he was in his thirties, forties, fifties, or sixties.

Sperm count in men is estimated to fall at a rate of 2.5 million per year. But with several hundred million sperm per ejaculation, men can arguably afford to lose some. The real question is how sperm of older men perform. The fact is, they swim slower, and more of them are deformed. They are also more likely to have chromosomal abnormalities, which is one reason why sperm banks draw their age limits at 40. The good news is that most lab tests fail to document an appreciable decrease in fertilizing potential associated with increasing male age.

Men themselves may also not perform as reliably as they age. With each succeeding decade after the late teen years, there is a distinct decrease in the ability of men to obtain erections easily. Men in their fifties may have to wait an entire day between sessions of intercourse to achieve an erection, compared to men in their twenties who can achieve another erection in 1 hour. Also, the force of a middle-aged man's ejaculation is not nearly as strong as a younger man's, and his sex drive wanes as his testosterone levels decline over time.

Because of the slight reproductive disadvantages in men age 35 and over, experts recommend the same basic strategies that can improve age-related pregnancy rates for women: Become an expert on ovulation timing and fertility-savvy sex, as chapters 12 and 13 discuss.

ACT NOW FOR MALE FERTILITY LATER

Unlike women, who've had it ingrained in them since puberty to have an annual gynecological exam, young men are rarely encouraged to schedule regular checkups with a urologist (the closest male health equivalent of a gynecologist). Guys don't get reminded by posters in public showers, movie stars on TV, and best friends to conduct self-examinations, either.

"Men don't generally meet a urologist until their first prostate exam at age 50. But I strongly encourage them to come to us—or their family doctor—any time they have a symptom or issue that concerns them," says Jean Fourcroy, M.D., a urologist and endocrinologist at Walter Reed Army Hospital and clinical assistant professor at the Uniformed Services University of Health Sciences in Bethesda, Maryland.

As is the case for women, early detection of male reproductive health concerns is critical. When testicular cancer is promptly diagnosed and treated, the sperm-generating capacity in at least one of the two testes can often be spared—along with the man's life. And what looks like a benign genital wart may be a harbinger for an otherwise symptomless STD or even penile cancer.

In the rest of this chapter, experts will outline some common health risks men need to be on the lookout for, as well as preventive actions they can take to avoid these problems from the start. If your significant other hasn't already been reading this book along with you, you might want to tag these pages for him and make sure he checks out the advice.

Watch Out for Infections

"When it comes to sexually transmitted infections, the signs for guys are usually less subtle than they are for women," says Dr. Metzger. "With chlamydia or gonorrhea, enough pus can come from the tip of the penis to fill a sock or sandwich bag. Syphilis and herpes produce sores and raw areas on the penis. For all these STDs, urinating may produce an excruciating burn." Anyone with common sense will dash into a public health clinic or see their doctor immediately, she remarks.

Infections of the prostate (prostatitis) or the tube connected to the testes (epididymitis) may be sexually transmitted, but they may also be lifestyle-related, autoimmune-based, or of unknown origin. (Infected seminal fluid often exhibits an array of bacterial and viral cultures, some rather obscure.) Symptoms include lower abdominal, testicular, or groin pain; difficulty urinating; general malaise; and, in their acute stage, fever and chills.

Antibiotics, along with anti-inflammatory medications, are the first line of treatment for infections of the male sexual organs. Here are some of the essentials of dodging infections to begin with.

Avoid "Pentagon syndrome." Because reflux of your own acidic urine may initiate an inflammatory reaction that starts off or prolongs an infection, Dr. Fourcroy cautions men against what she calls "Pentagon syndrome"—urinating in a rush. "When you void, it's very important that you take enough time to relax the urethra while you contract the bladder, rather than forcing it out," she explains.

Practice safe sex. Consistently using a male latex condom or a female condom with all sexual partners is the backbone of avoiding most sexually transmitted infections, including HIV. As reliable as condoms are, one particularly insidious infection, human papillomavirus (HPV) can be passed on with mere skin-to-skin contact. The most protective advice experts can offer for HPV is abstinence and limiting your number of sexual partners in life.

Spot Cancer and Other Red Flags

Prostate cancer deserves to be taken seriously. It's the most common cancer in men next to skin cancer, and it has a number of risk factors that can be reduced throughout life. But since prostate cancer is usually slow to develop and is most commonly diagnosed around the age of 70, a more immediate concern for men in their prime reproductive years is testicular and penile cancer.

Testicular cancer is the most common cancer among men ages 20 to 40. Cancer rates have doubled over the past 50 years in this sperm- and testosterone-generating organ. Fortunately, testicular cancer has a cure rate of 95 to 97 percent when found early, according to the American Medical Association. If you find a lump in your testicle, don't hesitate to have your doctor rule out a tumor (usually with an ultrasound). But don't panic—a testicular lump may also be a hernia, cyst, or an enlarged blood vessel. Although these conditions are relatively minor, they may still impair fertility when untreated.

Other symptoms of testicular cancer include enlargement or swelling of the testicles, an ache or sensation of heaviness in the lower abdomen, and even breast tenderness or enlargement from the hormones released by the tumor.

Since the tissues in the penis contain several types of cells, there are a number of varieties of penile cancer. By and large, penile cancer develops from flat, scalelike squamous cells on the surface of the skin. Since they are slow to develop, a man has a good chance of being cured. Superficial tumors can be treated with a laser, allowing preservation of both potency and fertility, says T. Ernesto Figueroa, M.D., clinical associate professor of urology at Jefferson University Medical College in Philadelphia. A guy should see a doctor to discuss any abnormal growths on the penis, including irritated or discolored patches of skin, or anything that looks like a wart or tiny cauliflower, according to the National Cancer Society.

In short, your life, your fertility, or both are at stake when it comes to genitourinary cancers. Here are some ways to reduce your risks.

Perform self-examinations. The American Cancer Society offers instructions for testicular self-exams. Although they can help any man catch a malignancy, self-exams are particularly important for those with a history of cryptorchidism (undescended testicles) or previous testicular cancer, or those with testicular cancer in their family. The best time to examine yourself is during or after a shower, when the skin of the scrotum is relaxed. Take a good 60 seconds to gently roll your fingers and thumbs along each of the testicles, searching for any hard lump or nodules (smooth, rounded masses). Also, take note of any changes in testicular shape or size. Immediately report any abnormalities to your doctor. "I encourage all men to do this on the first day of the month," says Dr. Figueroa.

You may also see or feel a large vein protruding out of your scrotum upon standing. If so, ask your doctor to check for a varicocele, a common obstruction that can impede the development of normal sperm, says Philip Werthman, M.D., a urologist specializing in male infertility and microsurgery who is director of the Center for Male Reproductive Medicine and chief of urology at Century City Hospital, both in Los Angeles. (See chapter 17 for more information on varicoceles.)

Wash well. The American Cancer Society reports that poor hygiene habits are associated with increased penile cancer risk—which helps explain why it occurs much more often in undeveloped countries. (Smegma, the material under the foreskin, may be to blame.) It's particularly important for uncircumcised men to retract their foreskin and clean the entire penis twice a day with soap and water, says Dr. Werthman. If your foreskin is constricted, your physician can make a small incision that makes it easier to retract.

Buy a vegetarian cookbook. Several studies suggest that diets high in animal fat may increase the risk of prostate cancer, while diets high in fruits, beans, vegetables, and whole grains may decrease the risk. The American Cancer Society recommends that all men limit their intake of animal products, especially red meat and high-fat dairy products. Lycopene in tomatoes is so prostate-friendly that the National Cancer Institute found that after eating a tomato-based meal every day for 3 weeks, even men with advanced prostate cancer were able to lower their levels of PSA (a marker for prostate cancer, prostatitis, and precancerous tumors).

Take E-protection. Fertility experts already promote antioxidants like vitamin E for their ability to help maintain sperm motility, and now it appears that vitamin E may protect against prostate cancer. The National Cancer Institute reports that men who took 50 milligrams of vitamin E daily for 5 to 8 years had 28 percent fewer cases of prostate cancer—and those men even smoked. (Of course, all men are urged to quit smoking to protect against cancer and sperm damage!)

Protect Yourself from Injury

Not only do sports make the hunter-warrior gender feel like the powerful, procreating forces that they are, but cardiovascular-challenging exercise protects men against multiple diseases, including cancer, and erectile dysfunction that could compromise their manhood. "The other side of the coin is that men, by their natures, will sustain blows and falls that can injure their gonads," says Dr. Metzger.

If you've sustained a testicular injury, don't be macho and continue to work or play. Stop what you're doing, lie down, and apply ice packs to relieve swelling and pain, advises Dr. Figueroa. "If the pain persists for more than 15 minutes, or if there is discoloration or swelling of the scrotum, seek immediate medical attention," he says.

Dr. Figueroa also cautions men that the best thing they can do to protect against genital injury is to wear an athletic cup and supporter while playing sports or doing strenuous exercise. "Make sure you have a good fit, and that you remember to also wear it as part of your pregame and prepractice routine," he says.

Biking poses another set of sport-related challenges to fertility, because cyclers' gonads are in nearly constant contact with the bicycle seat. When Austrian researchers took sensitive ultrasonographs of amateur mountain bikers, they discovered that 94 percent had some form of "microtrauma" in their sexual organs. (Only 16 percent of nonbikers had the same problems.) Although many of these abnormalities were relatively harmless cysts and calcifications, the injuries also included varicoceles and hydroceles (fertility-compromising obstructions). Not only is the constant vibration and impact of mountain biking hard on the internal structure of the male reproductive system, but bike saddles can compress the nerves and arteries that supply blood to the penis, potentially causing erectile dysfunction, Dr. Werthman points out.

Even road bicyclists navigating smoother surfaces than mountain bikers must take steps to protect against erectile dysfunction. After extensive research, Harvard University researchers concluded that men who ride 3 or more hours a week are 1.7 times more likely to develop erectile dysfunction than the general population. Few urologists discourage men from biking, though, saying the overall health benefits outweigh the risks. They do, however, offer a number of precautions that can make exercise easier on the family jewels.

Ride safe in the saddle. Rather than the classic long-nosed saddle that hits midline at the perineum (where the penile nerves are), experts recommend investing in an ergonomic saddle that distributes your weight more evenly. "I ride one myself," says Dr. Werthman. (The Specialized bike company makes a urologist-recommended Body Geometry Sport Saddle.) If you insist on riding a regular saddle, make sure it's gel-filled or padded and that you're sporting padded bike shorts. And be sure to adjust the seat so it's level or on a slight decline rather than upturned.

Take breaks. If you notice any tingling or numbness in your groin, get off the bike and walk around, advises Dr. Figueroa. Even if you feel fine, try to get off the bike every hour, experts say. (You don't necessarily have to feel any symptoms to have microtrauma or restricted bloodflow.) It's also recommended that you shift riding positions by standing occasionally.

Soften the blows. All cyclists should look for a bike with maximum suspension. The Austrian researchers suspected that full suspension could have reduced some of the microtrauma of men using only front-end suspension mountain bikes. Since it's not uncommon for bikers to fall against their top tube (the one under your crotch), men are also encouraged to use a bike with a slanting or step-through tube (guys need these more than women, for whom they are usually marketed!). At the very least, make sure the tube is no closer than 3 inches from your crotch when standing, and cover it with foam padding. Of course, a low-riding recumbent bike eliminate the risk altogether—so if you really want to be careful, it's a good option, says Dr. Werthman.

PART TWO

ACT NOW
TO
CONCEIVE
LATER

3

Beyond Basic Nutrition

Want to maximize your fertility? You may need to look no further than your dinner plate.

"Clearly, people who eat healthfully are healthier, and people who are healthier are more fertile," notes Machelle M. Seibel, M.D., director of the Fertility Center of New England in Dedham, Massachusetts, and author of *Soy Solutions for Menopause*. In fact, infertility is often the first sign that vital nutrients are missing from your diet or your partner's. Fortunately, changing how you eat is one of the simplest and most effective fertility-boosting strategies both of you can adopt. And the earlier you do it, the better.

That's because certain nutritional deficiencies may harm a developing fetus in the first few days of life—well before many women know they're pregnant. For instance, a lack of folic acid during the crucial fourth week of pregnancy (only about 2 weeks after your first missed period) can cause neural tube defects (NTDs) in a fetus, including spina bifida. Preventing health risks such as these is all the more reason why you and your partner should eat smart well *before* you conceive.

EAT CLOSE TO NATURE

Fostering fertility through diet is less about eating specific baby-making foods and more about eating balanced meals during your reproductive years that include as many natural foods as possible. By maximizing your health, a balanced diet based on natural, nutrient-rich foods will also optimize your fertility. For example, a healthful diet will improve the functioning of your immune system, which plays an important role in reproduction.

"Many young women's diets are really quite bad," notes Dr. Seibel. "These women are either overweight, or they're underweight because they want to fit into the right jeans. Often, they're not eating breakfast at all,

WHAT WORKED FOR US

HER NATURAL DIET LED TO BETTER HEALTH, INCREASED ENERGY— AND A BABY

Thirteen months after the birth of her daughter, Julia Indichova ran smack into her worst nightmare. A test revealed that her FSH (follicle-stimulating hormone) level was too high to produce fertilizable eggs. Doctors informed her that she and her husband wouldn't be able to have the second child they so desperately wanted.

In despair, Julia, then 42, turned to a string of New York fertility specialists, New Age gurus, and even a doctor of Chinese medicine—all without success. Then, 9 months into her quest to conceive, she had a sudden revelation inside a Manhattan health food store. "I thought, 'You've been going around trying to find someone to help you have a baby,'" she recalls. "'How about if you work on what you put into your body—something you can control?'"

First off, she stopped drowning her fertility frustrations in food. "Until then, I didn't think I could go on most days without cappuccino and a large piece of chocolate cake at 3 o'clock every afternoon," she says. "Many days I had no fruits or veggies at all. I decided to eliminate anything that was possibly harmful and focus on increasing life in my body so that my body would be able to produce life."

She simplified her diet—only fruit and juices until noon to cleanse her system,

so they're not getting B-complex vitamins or C vitamins from cereals and orange juice. They eat a lot of cheeseburgers and saturated fats and drink a lot of soda."

If you've been eating on autopilot lately, it's a good idea to break out a notebook and write down everything you eat for a few days. You might be surprised to see how few servings of fruits and vegetables you're getting—and how many processed or fatty foods you're consuming. "Charting what you eat for 2 or 3 days can be very eye-opening," notes Dr. Seibel.

One of the most basic—but also one of the most effective—changes you can make is to replace prepackaged foods in your diet with fresh, whole foods. "The closer you eat to nature, the better," advises M. Kelly

---

no meat except fish, only organic foods, more whole grains like millet and brown rice, no dairy products, and a glass of wheatgrass juice every day. Her husband, Ed Baum, a chef, revamped the family's meals with healthful dishes like tempeh with soy sauce, honey, and a touch of sesame oil; broccoli sautéed with olive oil and garlic; lentil soup; and adzuki-almond mousse for dessert.

Within 4 weeks, Julia noticed changes. The sinus headaches she'd suffered from for years cleared up. So did her rheumatism. She had more energy. Best of all, her menstrual cycles, which had been getting shorter, lengthened and the bloodflow grew brighter red and heavier. "It was an incredible boost for my sense of faith in myself," she remembers.

Eight months later, after Julia also incorporated yoga and visualization exercises into her daily routine, her body did what doctors had said was impossible: It conceived. In 1994, at age 44, she gave birth to her second daughter.

"I never really believed that what I ate could make such a difference until I saw it for myself," Julia admits.

For more information about Julia's fertility-enhancing diet, read her book, *Inconceivable: A Woman's Triumph over Despair and Statistics,* and visit her Web site at www.fertileheart.com.

Shanahan, M.D., author of *Your Over-35 Week-by-Week Pregnancy Guide* and chair of the obstetrics and gynecology department at Barton Memorial Hospital in South Lake Tahoe, California, where she is also the director of the Emerald Bay Center for Women's Health.

That means eating a mostly plant-based diet loaded with complex carbohydrates, such as fresh fruits, veggies, beans, and whole grains, and cutting back on processed grains, salty snacks, and sugary candies, cookies, and sodas—which are packed with simple carbohydrates that the body quickly converts to fat. In addition, diets high in simple carbs increase insulin levels, which can lead to polycystic ovary syndrome (PCOS), otherwise known as Stein–Leventhal disease, a condition known to interfere with fertility.

"A good diet should be 30 percent or fewer of calories from fat, and most of that should be unsaturated fats (like olive and other vegetable oils)," notes Yvonne Thornton, M.P.H., M.D., vice chairman and director of maternal–fetal medicine at Jamaica Hospital Medical Center in New York City.

About 50 grams of protein a day should work fine for most women, according to Ronald E. Burmeister, M.D., an infertility specialist with the Reproductive Health and Fertility Center in Rockford, Illinois, and assistant professor of obstetrics and gynecology at the University of Illinois College of Medicine at Rockford. "You can have a piece of meat or fish sometimes, but not at every meal."

Here are some specific recommendations for eating an optimum, fertility-enhancing diet.

Whole grains. Eat 6 to 11 servings of whole grains a day, including millet, brown rice, whole wheat, and oats. Whole grains are packed with nutrients necessary for optimum fertility, such as zinc, iron, and many B vitamins, including folate. Buy bread, crackers, pastas, and cereals made from these grains, too. Steer clear of white flour, white rice, and other refined grains, which offer little nutritional value because of processing.

Fruits and veggies. Produce should be fresh and eaten raw or slightly cooked. In fact, eating a salad every day with plenty of colorful, nutrient-rich veggies is a great way to boost fertility. Aim for three to five servings of veggies and two to four servings of fruit each day.

If you savor cooked vegetables, retain their nutrients by lightly steaming them. Leave on the nutrient-packed peels. Whenever possible, buy organic produce, which is grown without harmful pesticides that can hinder fertility and harm a growing fetus.

"If organic foods aren't available, be prepared to wash, wash, wash," notes Dr. Seibel. (For more on pesticides and environmental toxins that can rob your fertility, turn to chapter 9.)

Protein. Get two to three servings of meat, poultry, fish, beans, eggs, or

HOW MUCH IS A SERVING?

Follow this handy guide to determine what constitutes a serving of the foods you eat.

Food	1 Serving Equals . . .
Bread, cereal, rice, and pasta	1 slice of bread; 1 ounce of ready-to-eat cereal; or ½ cup of cooked cereal, rice, or pasta
Fruit	1 medium whole fruit; ½ cup chopped, cooked, or canned fruit; or ¾ cup of fruit juice
Vegetables	1 cup of raw leafy vegetables; ½ cup of other vegetables, cooked or chopped raw; or ¾ cup of vegetable juice
Meat, poultry, fish, dry beans, eggs, and nuts	2 to 3 ounces of cooked lean meat, poultry, or fish; ½ cup of cooked dry beans; 1 egg; or 2 tablespoons of nut butter or ⅓ cup of nuts
Milk, yogurt, and cheese	1 cup of milk or yogurt; 1½ ounces of natural cheese; or 2 ounces of processed cheese

nuts a day. Though meat is a top source of high-quality protein, its high fat and cholesterol content means you don't want to eat it at every meal. When you do decide to serve it, look for organic or free-range meats, raised without hormones, antibiotics, or pesticide-laden feeds.

Include fish in your diet once or twice a week, especially fatty, cold-water fish like salmon. Salmon is loaded with hormone-balancing omega-3 essential fatty acids (EFAs), which are lacking in many Western diets. But be aware that not all fish are equally good. Avoid swordfish, shark, king mackerel, and tilefish, which may contain methyl mercury that can harm your unborn baby's developing nervous system if you get pregnant. In addition, it's probably wise to eat tuna only once a week because of its relatively high mercury levels, cautions Howard Buttram, M.D., a board-certified expert in environmental and internal medicine who practices the Foresight Program for Preconception Care at The Woodlands Healing Research Center in Quakertown, Pennsylvania.

In place of meat, serve beans, such as lentils, adzuki beans, and chick-peas, as well as healthful nuts and seeds, which are good sources of fertility-fostering protein and EFAs.

Dairy. Look for organic milk, cheese, and other dairy products, and limit yourself to two to three servings a day.

Oils and fats. Go easy on fat, and avoid the hydrogenated vegetable oils with unnatural *trans* fats that are found in many prepared foods, such as cakes and cookies, and that contribute to insulin resistance and infertility. Instead, use cold-pressed unrefined vegetable oils, such as sesame, sunflower, canola, peanut, and extra virgin olive oil—all good sources of EFAs.

Fiber. To absorb the nutrients your body needs for reproduction, good digestion is key. Eating plenty of fiber, or roughage, assures that toxins and harmful bacteria are cleared out of your intestinal tract and good nutrients get in.

Eat a mix of soluble fiber, such as pectin found in fruit, and insoluble fiber, like wheat bran, which doesn't dissolve in water. Meals loaded with veggies, cereals, whole grain bread, nuts, seeds, and fruits, preferably with the hulls and peels left on, should provide all you need.

Water. Avoid constipation by drinking at least eight 8-ounce glasses of water every day. But don't save it all for mealtimes; too much liquid can dilute important digestive enzymes that help break down food.

BEWARE TOO MUCH OF A GOOD THING

Just because certain foods boost fertility doesn't mean that eating extra will further improve your conception odds. In fact, the opposite may be true.

For instance, animal foods—good sources of fertility-fostering protein and some essential nutrients—may actually raise estrogen levels and lead to fertility problems if eaten in excess. Indeed, endometriosis, an infertility-causing condition in which the uterine lining grows outside the uterus, may be related to a high-fat diet that includes a lot of red meat and dairy foods.

"Consuming animal-based essential fatty acids encourages the development of inflammatory prostaglandins, which are known to worsen endometriosis," Dr. Burmeister explains. "Women who switch to a vegetarian diet often see a lessening of symptoms."

Milk may be a good calcium source, but it can also wreak havoc on ovarian function. One study found that in populations where milk consumption is highest, women tend to be less fertile at older ages than non–milk-drinking women, and their drop-off in fertility is steeper. The culprit appears to be galactose, a sugar found in milk that many people can't digest, which somehow damages human eggs.

Fertility can also suffer if you have an allergy to milk or other dairy foods. Such allergies can thicken your cervical mucus and make it harder for sperm to reach an egg. Dairy allergies in men may thicken semen, diminishing the sperm's ability to move and fertilize eggs. Allergies to wheat and other gluten grains can have a similar effect.

If you have frequent heartburn, cramps, gas, or diarrhea and suspect that you have a food allergy, "keep a food diary and record everything you eat and how you felt afterward," advises Dr. Shanahan. "People who complain of feeling congested all the time may have a dairy allergy. If you feel lethargic or bloated after eating bread or pasta, you may have a wheat al-

THE DOWNSIDE OF SOY

From tempeh burgers to miso soup, soy has been hailed as a woman's panacea for everything from hot flashes to heart disease. But if you're planning to get pregnant, you may want to tone down your soy habit—at least the megadoses.

"Soy may affect female hormones," notes M. Kelly Shanahan, M.D., author of *Your Over-35 Week-by-Week Pregnancy Guide* and chair of the obstetrics and gynecology department at Barton Memorial Hospital in South Lake Tahoe, California, where she also runs the Emerald Bay Center for Women's Health. "In high doses, it may interfere with ovulation and implantation of an embryo."

Evidence that phytoestrogens—estrogen-mimicking compounds found in soy and other plants—can hinder female fertility comes mainly from animal studies. Captive cheetahs, California quails, and other species with diets high in phytoestrogens, such as daidzein and genistein, have reduced fertility.

No studies yet suggest that eating soy harms human fertility. But in 1999, Daniel R. Doerge, Ph.D., and Daniel M. Sheehan, Ph.D., top soy experts at the FDA, wrote a letter protesting the FDA's approval of soy protein to prevent heart disease because of its potential harm to other areas of the body, including estrogen-sensitive tissues in reproductive organs. The authors also noted that animal fetuses exposed in the womb to certain phytoestrogens display more reproductive "malformations," such as infertility. "During pregnancy in humans," they concluded, "isoflavones per se could be a risk factor for abnormal brain and reproductive tract development."

There's no need to completely eliminate tofu and other soy products if you're trying to conceive (though certain fertility problems might be helped by a no-soy diet), notes Toni Bark, M.D., director of integrative medicine at Advocate Good Shepherd Hospital's Health and Fitness Center in Barrington, Illinois, and medical director of the Center for Healing Arts in Glencoe, Illinois. In fact, soy is a good source of estriol, the main estrogen produced in pregnancy. But go easy on the big doses, she cautions.

"Infertility isn't a big problem in China or Japan, where women eat soy in regular amounts in their daily diet (such as miso soup with cubes of tofu in it)," Dr. Bark says. "But they're not eating gobs of soy powder in a protein shake every day. We don't know what the long-term effect of high doses is."

lergy. Stop eating these things for a while and see if the symptoms stop."

Be aware, however, that sometimes food allergy symptoms don't show up for 12 to 72 hours after you eat the food. In these cases, it can be difficult to identify the culprits with a food diary. If your diary doesn't seem to be giving you any clues about the offending foods, consider a visit to your doctor for skin or blood testing. You might also consider having a comprehensive stool analysis performed to see if there is evidence of dysbiosis (an imbalance of the good and bad bacteria and yeast) or other digestive enzyme deficiencies.

CONTROL YOUR BLOOD SUGAR

The amount of blood sugar, or glucose, circulating through your body can dramatically impact your fertility. Here's why.

After you eat, your blood sugar level starts to climb. Your body responds by producing insulin to shuttle the sugar into your cells for energy. When you eat plenty of complex carbohydrates, like whole grains, veggies, and fruits, which are low on the glycemic index (GI)—meaning they are digested and absorbed slowly—your blood sugar and insulin levels rise and fall gradually, remaining within the normal range. But when you dine on too many sugary foods and processed white breads and crackers (high-GI foods), your glucose and/or insulin levels shoot up faster and higher—often well above normal range.

Eventually, so much insulin is produced that your cells stop responding. This is called insulin resistance, and it lies at the root of a number of fertility-robbing conditions, including obesity, type 2 diabetes, syndrome X, and PCOS. (Check out chapters 5 and 16 for more on these insulin-related fertility disorders.) "Insulin resistance will alter hormones and affect ovulation," notes Toni Bark, M.D., director of integrative medicine at Advocate Good Shepherd Hospital's Health and Fitness Center in Barrington, Illinois, and medical director of the Center for Healing Arts in Glencoe, Illinois.

It's especially important to focus your meals on low-GI foods if you suffer from any condition linked to insulin resistance—such as hypoglycemia, a family history of diabetes, or being overweight—or are at risk for developing gestational diabetes during pregnancy. Even if you don't have any of these conditions, however, a diet based on low-GI foods is a good idea for both good general health and optimum fertility.

In addition, you might want to eat smaller meals more frequently, rather than three large meals a day, since this will keep your blood sugar levels more stable throughout the day. Exercising and losing weight (if you

FERTILITY VISIONARIES

Toni Bark, M.D.

Toni Bark, M.D., admits she found her infertility niche by accident. Trained in classical homeopathy—an approach that rights illness-causing imbalances in the body—she noticed about 6 years ago that other doctors were beginning to refer female patients to her for menstrual problems, hormonal disorders, and infertility. "I became known for balancing patients' hormones through nutritional approaches," she recalls. Soon, former patients were spreading the word.

Dr. Bark is director of integrative medicine at Advocate Good Shepherd Hospital's Health and Fitness Center in Barrington, Illinois, and medical director of the Center for the Healing Arts in Glencoe, Illinois. Infertility patients now account for one-fifth of her practice—and that number is growing. That's due, in part, to her impressive success rates. About 60 percent of her "infertile" patients eventually conceive after trying her hormone-balancing nutrition plan.

New patients meet with Dr. Bark for 2 hours to discuss their eating habits and lifestyle. Afterward, they undergo a series of tests to uncover hormone imbalances, including the ratio of estrogen to progesterone and luteinizing hormone (LH) to follicle-stimulating hormone (FSH).

No two fertility patients have the same imbalances, but many show similarities. "I see a lot of thin, semibulimic women who exercise too much and eat no fat. Their LH is usually suppressed," Dr. Bark says.

She also notices a direct connection between emotional health and hormone levels. "I see a lot of women originally from India who are in arranged

are over your ideal weight) also boost insulin sensitivity, as do drug thera-pies when lifestyle changes don't work.

STEER CLEAR OF BACTERIA AND FOOD ADDITIVES

Foods that are at risk for containing harmful bacteria should always be avoided during pregnancy and probably before conception, too. Here's a partial list of foods to bypass.

marriages and have an in-law in the house," she notes. "Their LH is elevated, often partly due to high-carbohydrate diets and resulting insulin resistance, and they've used up their progesterone by creating a lot of stress hormones as they suppress so much of themselves."

Every patient follows basic dietary strategies—all are urged to munch plenty of veggies and fruits and eat up to 70 percent of their food either raw or slightly cooked—but each also follows a customized nutrition plan. Women with too much strong estrogen, for instance, may be encouraged to sprinkle 3 tablespoons of ground flaxseed (rich in essential fatty acids, or EFAs, and lignans) on oat bran or in orange juice to help metabolize their estrogen into weaker metabolites. Or they could take soy or get indole-3-carbinol from cruciferous vegetables for the same purpose. Women on ultra-low-fat diets are encouraged to eat more healthy fats, like those in avocados, walnuts, and olive oil and also usually begin a regimen of EFA supplements.

"I try to address the underlying imbalance on an individual basis," Dr. Bark notes.

Contact information: Contact Dr. Bark at the Center for the Healing Arts, 650 Vernon Avenue, Glencoe, IL 60022. Her phone number there is (847) 835-6207. At Advocate Good Shepherd Hospital, call (847) 620-4565. Dr. Bark also provides treatment for patients outside the Chicago area via phone consultation.

Sushi. Raw fish may contain infection-causing parasites that can lead to miscarriages.

Soft, unpasteurized cheeses. That includes brie, Roquefort, Camembert, feta, and blue cheese. All may contain *Listeria*, a bacteria linked to stillbirths and miscarriages.

Smoked lunchmeats. Not only do smoked lunchmeats sometimes harbor *Listeria*, but they are loaded with nitrates, cancer-causing food additives.

While food additives aren't linked specifically to infertility or birth defects, they are chemicals and may play a role in asthma, headaches, childhood hyperactivity, and other as-yet-undetermined disorders. Avoiding artificial colors, sweeteners, flavor enhancers such as monosodium glutamate (MSG), and preservatives, such as sulphites and benzoates, is no easy feat. About 75 percent of a typical Western diet is composed of processed foods, and most of us eat 8 to 10 pounds of food additives every year.

The best approach is vigilance. That means reading food labels and choosing mostly natural and organic products. Remember: Mother Nature knows best when it comes to the best diet for mothers-to-be. Eat as close to nature as possible.

SUPPLEMENT WISELY

For women who aren't planning on becoming pregnant in the future, supplements provide an extra bit of nutritional "insurance" against a diet that might not always be optimal. But if you *are* planning a pregnancy in the near or even not-so-near future, supplements are a vital part of your self-care. If you and your partner haven't been taking vitamin supplements all along, now's the time for both of you to start.

For Women

Start taking a prenatal multivitamin with minerals—either an over-the-counter or prescription brand—at least 3 months before you plan to get pregnant so your body has time to rev up its fertility and stockpile baby-making nutrients, recommends Dr. Shanahan.

While there's still a lot of research to be done to determine which vitamins and minerals actually boost fertility, recommendations can be inferred from the amounts suggested for pregnancy. Here are some of the top nutrients that either enhance fertility or improve pregnancy outcomes, as recognized by Dr. Seibel in his studies. (For a more complete list of vital nutrients, see "Quick Reference: What Women Need before and during Pregnancy" on page 64.) Be aware that some of the dosages recommended below exceed the Dietary Reference Intakes (DRIs) for pregnancy, which are minimum requirements. Be sure to talk with your doctor to determine the dosage that's right for you.

Folic acid. Besides raising the risk of neural tube defects (NTDs) in the first few weeks of pregnancy, a deficiency in this B vitamin also increases your chances of miscarrying and having a low-birth-weight baby. Eat plenty of foods rich in folate (the natural form of this vitamin), such as spinach, turnips, mustard greens, citrus fruits, beans, lentils, and black-eyed peas, and take between 400 and 800 micrograms of folic acid daily. (If you previously had a child with a neural tube defect, talk with your doctor about increasing this amount to between 1,000 and 4,000 micrograms.)

Vitamin B_{12}. This vitamin is found in foods containing animal protein, such as meat, fish, and eggs, and is vital for normal cell division (that's important for your unborn baby's growth). If you eat these foods regularly, you're probably getting the recommended amount for pregnant women, 2.6 micrograms daily. If not, make sure your vitamin contains enough. (*Note:* If your doctor discovers that you're deficient in vitamin B_{12}, she may recommend sublingual pills, nasal sprays, or injections, since these may be absorbed better than standard B_{12} supplements.)

Vitamin B_6. Many women are deficient in this vital nutrient for metabolizing proteins and carbohydrates. Because pregnancy further deletes stores, start taking 2 milligrams a day. An added bonus: Once you become pregnant, vitamin B_6 is a natural antinausea remedy.

Vitamin C. This key antioxidant keeps your body, including your reproductive organs, running efficiently and is found in fresh fruits and veggies. During pregnancy, 80 to 85 milligrams is recommended daily, but Dr.

QUICK REFERENCE: WHAT WOMEN NEED BEFORE AND DURING PREGNANCY

Check out the following chart from the National Academy of Sciences and the National Institutes of Health Office of Dietary Supplements for specific daily dosages of the vitamins and minerals that are essential before and during pregnancy. The amounts are broken down by age group. Bear in mind that the dosages listed are the minimum requirements, but many women may need more. Talk to your doctor or nutritionist about what's right for you.

	Dietary Reference Intakes (DRIs) for Pregnancy		
Nutrient	Less Than 19 Years	19 to 30 Years	31 to 50 Years
Vitamin A	770 RE	770 RE	770 RE
Vitamin B_6	1.9 mg	1.9 mg	1.9 mg
Vitamin B_{12}	2.6 mcg	2.6 mcg	2.6 mcg
Vitamin C	80 mg	85 mg	85 mg
Vitamin D	5 mcg	5 mcg	5 mcg
Vitamin E	15 mg (22 IU)	15 mg (22 IU)	15 mg (22 IU)
Biotin	30 mcg	30 mcg	30 mcg
Calcium	1,300 mg	1,000 mg	1,000 mg
Choline	450 mg	450 mg	450 mg
Fluoride	3 mg	3 mg	3 mg
Folic acid	600 mcg	600 mcg	600 mcg
Iron	27 mg	27 mg	27 mg
Magnesium	400 mg	350 mg	360 mg
Niacin	18 mg	18 mg	18 mg
Pantothenic acid	6 mg	6 mg	6 mg
Phosphorus	1,250 mg	700 mg	700 mg
Riboflavin	1.4 mg	1.4 mg	1.4 mg
Selenium	60 mcg	60 mcg	60 mcg
Thiamin	1.4 mg	1.4 mg	1.4 mg
Zinc	12 mg	11 mg	11 mg

Burmeister advises taking 1,000 milligrams for extra insurance. If you currently smoke or take birth control pills, you may need more. Talk with your doctor.

Vitamin A. An essential antioxidant, vitamin A not only protects mucous membranes—including those in the reproductive tract—from infection, but it also safeguards your unborn baby against cell mutations and birth defects, such as eye defects. Most prenatal vitamins offer vitamin A in the form of beta-carotene, which is safer because the body excretes what's not needed. For pregnancy, a minimum of 770 retinol equivalents (2,565 IU) is recommended. Don't exceed 10,000 IU, which can lead to birth defects.

Vitamin E. Discovered in 1922 during rat experiments, this powerful antioxidant contains tocopherols, a Greek word meaning "to bear children." Scientists found that rats without vitamin E in their diets became infertile. Fertility was restored by adding it back in. More recent studies suggest that vitamin E may reduce age-related ovulation decline.

Vitamin E has been shown to relieve high blood pressure in pregnancy (called preeclampsia) and the complications that can result, such as kidney impairment and premature delivery. Dr. Burmeister recommends 400 IU a day.

Choline. Fetuses that don't get enough choline may be born with impaired attention and memory. Eggs, liver, peanuts, and many meats are rich sources of this vital nutrient. If your diet is low in these foods, take the recommended amount for pregnancy of 450 milligrams daily.

Iron. Anemia affects between 10 and 20 percent of American women of reproductive age and often leads to pregnancy complications. Because a developing fetus uses so much of its mother's iron, your need increases dramatically in pregnancy. Dr. Seibel recommends taking 30 milligrams of elemental iron a day.

Zinc. Because iron can interfere with the absorption of zinc, Dr. Seibel advises supplementing with 15 milligrams a day. Low zinc levels can lead to birth defects and low birth weights.

Calcium. A growing baby increases your calcium requirement by 200 to 300 milligrams a day. Try to get between 1,000 and 1,300 milligrams a day before and during pregnancy, either by eating dairy products or by taking calcium citrate to make up the difference.

Selenium. Deficiency has been shown to reduce egg production and increase birth defects in animals. Take 60 micrograms a day.

Magnesium. If you are at risk for having a low-birth-weight or premature baby, taking prenatal magnesium may reduce the risk for cerebral palsy and mental retardation. Pregnant women over the age of 19 should consume 350 to 360 milligrams of magnesium daily. Magnesium may also reduce your chance of developing preeclampsia.

Essential fatty acids. No daily requirements have been established for omega-3 and omega-6 EFAs before and during pregnancy, but Dr. Shanahan advises getting a good balance mostly from the foods you eat. A proper balance is particularly important for regulating reproductive hormones and boosting fetal brain development.

Because a typical Western diet is usually high in omega-6s, found abundantly in common vegetable oils, focus on decreasing your intake of vegetable oils and boosting your intake of the less abundant omega-3s. In addition to eating cold-water fish such as salmon twice a week, eat more green leafy veggies and beans. Flaxseed is another excellent source of omega-3s and is available in your health food store as an oil (good for salads) or as a supplement, if you can't get enough in your daily diet. Other good sources include fish oil and borage oil capsules, both of which are also available in health food stores.

For Men

Dr. Seibel suggests that men take a multivitamin with all the B vitamins. In addition to that, there are a few other nutrients to consider, particularly if your sperm counts or motility are low. Consult with your doctor or nutritionist first for specific recommendations.

Folic acid. Not only does folic acid prevent NTDs during pregnancy, but it also appears to boost sperm counts. Dr. Burmeister recommends 400 micrograms a day.

Vitamin C. Deficiency of this vital antioxidant may reduce sperm counts

PROMISING FERTILITY BOOSTERS FOR MEN

Though the jury's still out on the specific fertility-boosting effects of many vitamins and minerals for men, the following ones have shown promise, notes Melanie Koeman, N.D., a naturopathic doctor at Jocelyn Centre for Natural Fertility Management and Holistic Medicine in Sydney, Australia.

Nutrient	Recommended Therapeutic Dose (per Day)
Vitamin B_{12}	500 to 1,500 mcg
Vitamin C with bioflavonoids	1,000 to 3,000 mg
Vitamin E	500 to 1,000 IU
Arginine	3,000 mg
Beta-carotene	6 to 20 mg
Carnitine	1,200 mg
Coenzyme Q_{10} (lipid capsule)	30 to 100 mg
Folic acid	400 mcg
Histidine	800 mg
Selenium	200 to 400 mcg
Zinc	25 to 50 mg

and motility (the sperm's ability to move). Take at least 1,000 milligrams a day, advises Dr. Burmeister.

Vitamin E. Another key antioxidant, vitamin E improves sperm motility and its ability to fertilize eggs. Take at least 400 IU a day.

Selenium. This nutrient also boosts overall sperm function. Try 200 to 400 micrograms daily.

Zinc. Take 25 to 50 milligrams a day to raise sperm counts and boost testosterone levels.

USE CAUTION WITH HERBS

Just because something comes from a plant doesn't mean it isn't also a powerful drug. In fact, many of the drugs that are prescribed by physicians were derived from herbs. If you and your partner are ready to conceive, you'll want to closely evaluate the herbs you use—including herbal teas. At the very least, check with your doctor or herbalist first.

"Have a list of everything you take and what you want to know when you visit your doctor, so you don't forget anything," suggests Dr. Seibel. Still, be aware that, with the exception of just a few select herbs, your doctor will probably advise you to give up herbal remedies before and during pregnancy.

Here is the short list of herbs that are generally considered safe for use before and during pregnancy.

* Lemon balm (stimulates digestion and cleanses your system of toxins)

* Raspberry leaf (uterine tonic that can strengthen your reproductive system)

* Dandelion (but not from your yard if you spray with fertilizers and weed killers)

* Echinacea (Though this herb is generally considered safe, check with your doctor before using it, and don't use it in combination with goldenseal, which can induce abortions.)

Keep your distance from the following herbs, all of which can be dangerous during pregnancy, says Dr. Shanahan.

* Fresh ginger (can cause miscarriage, if taken in extremely high amounts)

* *Ginkgo biloba* (blood thinner that might cause bleeding in early pregnancy)

* *Panax notoginseng* (this type of ginseng may raise blood pressure; other varieties of ginseng are considered safe during pregnancy)

* Ma huang or ephedra (may boost blood pressure)

* Pennyroyal (can induce abortions)

4

Good Advice for Bad Habits

Smoking. Too much alcohol. Excess caffeine. Illegal drugs. We're probably not creating any headlines by proclaiming that these are all known health hazards. But what many women aren't aware of is that these bad habits can also diminish their conception odds.

Weaning yourself and your partner off these fertility robbers is one of the smartest and least costly strategies you can adopt to keep both of your reproductive systems in optimum shape until you're ready to conceive—whether that's now or not for another 10 years. And cutting out bad habits may also ensure that you have an easier pregnancy and a healthier baby, too.

"You probably can't extend your fertility, but you can make the most of the fertile life span you have," notes Ronald F. Feinberg, M.D., Ph.D., associate adjunct professor of obstetrics and gynecology at Yale University School of Medicine and in vitro fertilization medical director of Reproductive Associates of Delaware in Newark. To optimize your fertile life span, you need to ditch habits that harm your health. After all, less robust general health often means a corresponding decrease in fertility.

There's good news, too, if you're currently trying for a baby but haven't yet succeeded. Curbing toxic habits now may offer you and your partner just the fertility boost you need to conceive. "Giving your body the best chance to do what it wants to do through a healthier lifestyle goes a long way toward a healthy, happy pregnancy," says reproductive endocrinologist Mark Perloe, M.D., medical director of Georgia Reproductive Specialists in Atlanta and author of *Miracle Babies and Other Happy Endings.*

TOSS THE PACK

Cigarette smoking is one habit you and your partner will want to lose fast. Evidence of its devastating impact on both female and male reproductive health is overwhelming and undeniable.

"Smoking is bad no matter which way you look at it," notes Robert L. Barbieri, M.D., chairman of the obstetrics and gynecology department at Brigham and Women's Hospital in Boston, an obstetrics and gynecology professor at Harvard Medical School, and coauthor of *Six Steps to Increased Fertility.*

Old before Their Time

Perhaps the most convincing reason for women to kick the habit sooner rather than later comes from ample evidence showing that harmful compounds in tobacco smoke actually age the ovaries and kill eggs. In other words, indulging your nicotine cravings might just throw you into menopause years before the average age of 51.

What's more, the longer you've smoked and the earlier you started, the greater the impact on your fertility. One study found that women who began lighting up before age 18 were three times more likely to enter menopause before their 40th birthday than nonsmokers. Add to that smoke-related genetic damage inflicted on eggs, as well as a diminished ability to make estrogen, and your fertility odds drop even further. "A 35-year-old woman who smokes probably has the ovaries of about a 40-year-old," notes Dr. Barbieri.

If you're currently undergoing infertility treatment, smoking may also cut your success rate. Women pursuing in vitro fertilization have been shown to lower their chance of pregnancy by nearly one-third if they smoke.

Clearing the Air for Moms-to-Be

When it comes to smoking, the fertility burden appears to fall more on a woman's shoulders than on a man's. But that doesn't mean guys should feel free to light up. The evidence may be murkier, but a link between male smoking and diminished fertility does exist, particularly among men who smoke one to two packs a day. Effects include fewer sperm, a lower proportion of motile sperm, reduced levels of the male hormone testosterone, and genetic damage to sperm that can cause birth defects. What's more, damage shows up early, even in male teenagers who smoke.

If for no other reason, men should give up cigarettes to create a smoke-free environment for their partners. Exposure to secondhand smoke has been shown to diminish a woman's odds of conceiving within 6 months. In fact, both you and your partner should avoid secondhand smoke whenever possible, since passive smoke inhalation is believed to harm male and female reproductive health almost as much as active smoking does.

No Time Like the Present

"The day you stop smoking, you will prevent any further damage to your eggs," notes Stephen G. Somkuti, M.D., Ph.D., director of the in vitro fertilization program at Abington Memorial Hospital in Pennsylvania and assistant clinical professor at Jefferson Medical College in Philadelphia. Granted, you can't reverse the harm already inflicted—women are born with all the eggs they'll ever have—but you can "boost your chances of pregnancy a few percentage points," he says. Indeed, data show that women who are ex-smokers often achieve fertility rates similar to those of women who have never smoked, even if they quit within a year of trying for a baby.

Men have more leeway in terms of reversing smoke damage to sperm

WHAT WORKED FOR US
BANNING THE BUTTS BRINGS A WELCOME SURPRISE

When Deb Loman* finally visited a fertility doctor after trying to get pregnant for years, one thing he suggested was to quit smoking. Her half-a-pack-a-day habit didn't seem like an impediment to pregnancy, but when she learned that even small amounts of nicotine could cut fertility, she was willing to try.

The next year and a half was a roller-coaster ride. Deb tried fertility medications, artificial insemination, and in vitro fertilization—all the while struggling to kick the habit cold turkey. "I tried to take my mind off smoking by being busy—usually by taking the dog for a walk," she recalls. "We both got a lot of exercise."

Months into treatment, Deb finally reined in her nicotine urge. But by that time, discouragement was setting in. After her fourth unsuccessful in vitro attempt, she realized that at 37, she might never get pregnant. "I told my husband, 'I can't do this anymore—it's too heartbreaking,' and we started checking out adoption," she says.

Shortly afterward, in November, the couple went on a Caribbean cruise to relax and gear themselves up for the adoption process. The vacation—and the decision to end the frustrating in vitro treatments—did a lot to relieve the stress they both were feeling. Once back home in suburban Philadelphia, Deb started feeling sick to her stomach and tired. Right before Christmas she called her doctor, who suggested she come in for a blood test. That afternoon he phoned with some astounding news. She was pregnant.

"I was totally floored," Deb recalls. "I went out and bought a home pregnancy test because I didn't believe it."

Now in her fifth month, Deb is convinced that letting go of stress and giving up her smoking habit are the reasons she finally conceived. "To me it's a miracle," she says.

* Name has been changed for confidentiality

because new sperm are produced every day. But because the average sperm requires 72 to 90 days to mature, quitting several months before trying to conceive will ensure that all new sperm are in prime shape.

Kicking the habit in advance also ensures that you won't unknowingly become pregnant while you or your partner is still smoking. Babies born to mothers who smoke during pregnancy tend to have lower birth weights and a host of birth defects, such as cleft palates, learning difficulties, and hyperactivity. Likewise, babies with smoking fathers are also born with more birth defects. In addition, smokers have nearly twice the risk of miscarriage.

Nix the Nicotine with These Strategies

The best way to beat your nicotine need is to use drug therapy in combination with group or individual counseling. Quitting cold turkey is an option but can be hard going when willpower flags and you have no one to turn to for encouragement and support. The FDA has approved five medications, including nicotine gum and the nicotine patch, that may double your chances of stopping permanently. Talk to your doctor about trying one of these, as well as finding a good smoking-cessation program at your local hospital or health center.

Here are some other tips to help you beat the tobacco temptation.

* Set a quit date. When the day comes, throw out all cigarettes and ashtrays in your home, car, and workplace.

* Don't let people smoke in your home, and ask family, friends, and coworkers to support you by not smoking around you. If both you and your partner are smokers, try making a pact that you'll quit together.

* Change your routine and avoid triggers that cause you to smoke. For instance, if you like to smoke immediately after breakfast, eat someplace new, whether that's a different coffee shop or simply a different room in your house. If stress is usually your cue to light up, take a hot bath or go for a walk instead.

* If you smoke because it gives you something to do with your hands and satisfies an oral fixation, try to transition to healthier substitutes. Gum, mints, carrots, tea, or water can serve as alternatives.

For more tips, call the American Lung Association at (800) LUNGUSA or visit www.lungusa.org.

To avoid secondhand smoke, check out the following strategies.

* Ask all visitors and family members to smoke outdoors instead of in your home. Allow no exceptions—remember, it's your house, so you get to make the rules, no matter who grumbles about them!

* If your company doesn't have a secondhand smoke policy, help establish one. Separating smokers and nonsmokers in one area, like a cafeteria, can reduce your exposure, but you'll still be exposed to recirculated smoke and smoke that drifts into nonsmoking spots. A better plan is to prohibit smoking indoors altogether or to limit smoking to specially designed rooms that keep smoke from escaping.

* In restaurants, ask to be seated in nonsmoking areas as far from smokers as possible, or visit only those restaurants that prohibit smoking altogether.

POP THE CORK IN MODERATION

A romantic night of baby-making conjures up images of soft music and champagne. But before you and your partner pour the bubbly—or any alcoholic drink—consider this: Depending on how much and how often you drink, liquor can reduce your fertility and your partner's.

"Conventional wisdom says moderation in everything," notes Dr. Somkuti. "That goes for alcohol, too."

Nearly three-quarters of American women report drinking alcohol at least once in a while; one-quarter consume more than four drinks a week. (Researchers define a drink as 12 ounces of beer, 5 ounces of wine, or 1.5 ounces of hard liquor.) While doctors now tout the benefits of a glass of red wine a day to help ward off conditions like heart disease and high cholesterol, the data on drinking and conception is still mixed.

On one hand, a recent Danish study of more than 39,000 pregnant women found that those who drank a moderate amount of alcohol (fewer than two drinks a day) in the months prior to conception didn't have a harder time getting pregnant than nondrinkers, perhaps because the alcohol helped the women feel more relaxed. In fact, women who didn't drink at all actually had slightly longer wait times than moderate drinkers. "Some of the latest articles suggest that moderate use of alcohol may actually enhance metabolism—and anything that enhances metabolism and insulin action may improve fertility," adds Dr. Feinberg.

Other studies, however, suggest that drinking and conception don't mix. For instance, one found that women who drank more than 8 drinks

WHAT WORKED FOR US

SHE BEAT HER DOCTOR'S DIAGNOSIS BY OVERHAULING HER LIFESTYLE

Like many women, Janine Francolini waited until her career and marriage were solid and thriving before trying for a family. When she turned 31, the time finally seemed right, and she and her husband launched into baby-making.

Two and a half years later, she still wasn't pregnant. "We tried infertility treatment, but the doctor eventually said I'd never get pregnant because I was in premature menopause," she recalls.

Unable to accept her doctor's diagnosis, Janine, a nursery school admissions director in Manhattan, did some research and decided to take matters into her own hands. Her first move was to drop some bad habits linked to infertility. That meant forgoing her three-cup-a-day coffee habit and the three to five glasses of wine she enjoyed each week. Her husband also cut down on his alcohol consumption.

In addition, Janine started taking yoga classes three times a week and adopted a fertility-boosting dietary plan, which involved cutting out refined sugars and dairy products and buying mostly organic foods, including loads of fresh fruits and veggies. Typical meals included nothing but fruit for breakfast, then lunches and dinners of fish or chicken, nuts, hummus, and lots of veggies.

"After making these changes, I had so much more energy—I felt great," she says. The result? Within months, she was pregnant and now has a healthy young son.

Although Janine has since resumed drinking coffee and an occasional glass of wine, she's convinced that healthier living is the reason she got pregnant. In fact, she's about to do it all again. "I'm getting revved up for the next baby," she admits.

per week were at slightly greater risk of infertility linked with not ovulating properly or with endometriosis, a condition in which fragments of the uterine lining migrate to other parts of the pelvic cavity, resulting in inflammation and the inability to conceive.

Research on male drinking suggests that heavy—although not moderate—drinking can cut testosterone and sperm production and lead to impotence.

The Bottom Line . . .

"If you already have a drink a day, there's probably no downside in terms of fertility," notes Dr. Feinberg. "But if you don't already drink, I'm not recommending that you start."

As you begin trying for a baby, you and your partner should try to limit alcohol. For women, your best bet is no more than four drinks per week, says Dr. Barbieri. Men may have more latitude, but moderation is still key.

For the biggest reproductive boost possible, some experts recommend closing up the liquor cabinet altogether at least 4 months before trying to conceive. Likewise, couples who are having trouble conceiving should consider a moratorium on alcohol. Avoiding alcohol in the months before conception also ensures that you won't unwittingly expose your unborn child to alcohol if you become pregnant without knowing it. Exposure to alcohol in the womb can cause a host of physical and mental defects in your baby, including brain and heart malformations. In fact, no amount of alcohol has been found to be safe during pregnancy. In other words, better to be safe than sorry.

Finally, if you believe either you or your partner has a drinking problem, talk to your doctor about treatment programs near you or look in the blue pages of your phone book, under "Guide to Human Services." For brochures on alcohol abuse and 24-hour treatment referral information in your area, you can call the U.S. Substance Abuse and Mental Health Services Administration (SAMHSA) at (800) 662-HELP. Or check out their online Treatment Facility Locator at www.findtreatment.samhsa.gov.

THE CAFFEINE CONNECTION

If your idea of morning heaven is multiple trips to the coffeemaker, you may need to rethink your A.M. priorities for peak fertility. The fact is, the less caffeine you consume, the better your chances of getting pregnant. There's little evidence that caffeine impacts male fertility, but guys shouldn't grab too many morning refills either. "I'm not telling patients to get rid of caffeine altogether," notes Dr. Feinberg, "but several months before trying to conceive, women should start weaning themselves off it."

While the caffeine–infertility connection isn't as compelling as the data on smoking and alcohol, small but significant links do exist—especially for women who drink more than 250 milligrams of caffeine daily in coffee (8 ounces of brewed coffee contains 135 milligrams) or get an equivalent amount from other sources, such as chocolate, colas, tea, and painkillers.

First, caffeine causes the liver to release glycogen, which is turned into glucose. In response, your insulin levels increase, says Deborah Metzger, M.D., Ph.D., medical director of Helena Women's Health in San Jose, California, and medical advisor to this book. Elevated insulin levels have been implicated as a common factor in infertility. "Drinking a cup of a caffeinated beverage is like eating a glazed doughnut," she notes.

In addition, caffeine is believed to hamper fertility by boosting estrogen production or slashing estrogen metabolism or both, thereby upsetting the delicate hormonal balance needed for normal ovulation and pregnancy.

The greatest impact seems to be on women who consume more than 500 milligrams of caffeine daily. In one study, 23 percent of couples with female partners who drank five or more cups of coffee a day hadn't conceived after 9½ months, compared with 16 percent of couples in which the female partners didn't drink coffee. Consider also that five or more cups of coffee a day during pregnancy can raise your risk of miscarriage.

A Safe Limit?

"For couples attempting conception, it's probably okay for the woman to drink two cups of coffee a day or less," notes Dr. Barbieri. If you have

CAFFEINE HIGH

Think caffeine, and you may immediately picture a large cup of coffee or a double espresso, but as you'll see, caffeine also pops up in some less obvious beverages, foods, and even medications.

Product	Caffeine Content (mg)
Brewed coffee (8 oz)	135
Instant coffee (8 oz)	95
Decaffeinated coffee (8 oz)	5
Brewed tea (8 oz)	50
Green tea (8 oz)	30
Mountain Dew soft drink (12 oz)	55.5
Diet Coke (12 oz)	46.5
Sunkist Orange Soda (12 oz)	42
Pepsi-Cola (12 oz)	37.5
Hershey's Special Dark chocolate bar	31
Hershey's milk chocolate bar	10
Excedrin pain medication (2 tablets)	130
NoDoz maximum strength (1 tablet)	200

been trying to follow a low-glycemic diet, however, it's probably best to abstain from caffeine altogether.

Also, if you've been having trouble conceiving, halting your caffeine habit altogether might just sharpen your reproductive edge. "I personally believe that any amount ingested per day adds up over a lifetime," notes Dr. Somkuti.

Begin reining in caffeine consumption by looking at everything you eat and drink. You may be getting more than you think (see "Caffeine High").

If coffee is your main caffeine vice, try switching to decaffeinated coffee or tea (nonherbal decaffeinated tea is available in supermarkets and via the Internet). If you're a serious java junkie, you may want to wean yourself off the brew slowly, decreasing your consumption by half a cup per week to avoid withdrawal headaches. Other alternatives include mixing half decaf and half regular or making every other cup decaf.

DRUGS AND PREGNANCY: A DEADLY MIX

When it comes to illegal drug use and pregnancy, there is no room for ambiguity: If you use illegal drugs, even recreationally, you need to take every possible precaution *not* to get pregnant. Regular use of almost any drug during pregnancy, including marijuana, heroin, cocaine, and methamphetamines, can cause miscarriage, premature labor, and low birth weights. Cocaine can also cause placental abruption, separation of the placenta from the uterus wall. Furthermore, taking drugs such as cocaine or heroin late in pregnancy may cause your baby to be born addicted.

The evidence is still scant on whether marijuana, cocaine, and other illegal drugs diminish fertility, but experts agree that they have no place in healthy baby-making. "If there's an issue of substance abuse, you shouldn't be trying to get pregnant," emphasizes Dr. Perloe.

Marijuana has been shown to decrease testosterone levels, lower sperm counts, and slash sex drive in men. Cocaine is also known to inhibit male fertility. "There's not much data on female fertility and drug use," notes Dr. Somkuti, "but certainly women shouldn't use drugs either."

Even certain over-the-counter and prescription drugs, like aspirin, ibuprofen, and medications to control high blood pressure, can act as fertility robbers or harm your growing baby if you're already pregnant. In fact, it's a good idea to consult with your doctor at least 3 months before trying to conceive to see if you can stop taking your prescription drugs or can switch to a medication that is safer to fertility and a potential fetus. And once you're pregnant, always check with your doctor before taking any drug, even an over-the-counter one. (See chapter 10 for more information on how common medications can harm fertility.)

If either you or your partner has an addiction problem, talk to your doctor about substance abuse treatment programs in your area or check the blue pages of your phone directory under "Guide to Human Services."

5

Sizing Up Weight and Fitness Factors

Working up a sweat *outside* the bedroom can have a positive impact on what happens *inside* it. After all, regular workouts not only boost your general health, but they also keep your reproductive organs in prime shape for baby-making. Ditto for your partner. With frequent workouts, you'll both feel better physically and mentally, which means a rise in libido. Plus, exercise helps you maintain a fertility-friendly weight by burning excess calories and body fat, while also preparing your body for the rigors of childbirth.

The trick, though, is finding just the right fitness formula. Either too much exercise or too little can impair fertility, particularly in women. "I believe moderation is the key," notes Ronald F. Feinberg, M.D., Ph.D., in vitro fertilization medical director of Reproductive Associates of Delaware in Newark and associate adjunct professor of obstetrics and gynecology at Yale University School of Medicine. "Exercising 3 to 7 hours a week will generally enhance metabolic function, self-esteem, and overall health. It also reduces stress—all positives for reproductive function."

If you're planning to get pregnant and exercise isn't part of your health regimen, now's the time to dust off those sneakers. "I recommend starting with 20 to 30 minutes of walking a few times a week if you haven't exercised before," says reproductive endocrinologist Mark Perloe, M.D., medical director of Georgia Reproductive Specialists in Atlanta and author of *Miracle Babies and Other Happy Endings*. Other fertility-boosting activities include jogging, tennis, swimming, weight machines, dancing, and anything else that gets you up and moving—as long as you don't go overboard.

TONE BACK IF YOU'RE A FITNESS FANATIC

Too much of a good thing can actually rob you and your partner of fertility. Overzealous exercise can decrease brain messages to the female reproductive organs, causing them to stop functioning properly. Women who exercise a lot—we're talking marathon runners, ballerinas, and aerobics addicts—often have menstrual irregularities and may even stop menstruating altogether, a condition known as hypothalamic amenorrhea. Eating disorders like bulimia and anorexia nervosa have a similar effect on reproduction.

But even if you aren't pounding the pavement every morning at dawn, you may still be overdoing it. Studies show that more than 1 hour of strenuous aerobic activity daily or more than 10 miles of running a week can reduce your conception odds. "If you've been into exercise all along, I suggest toning your workouts down before conception to a level where you can still talk and aren't winded," advises Dr. Perloe.

Men have greater latitude when it comes to fitness, but too many workouts by the male partner can also decrease a couple's conception odds by cutting sperm production. The 10-mile-a-week rule is probably a good idea for potential dads-to-be, too.

In addition, men who use androgenic steroids for bodybuilding should either stop or talk to their doctor. "Misuse or abuse of steroids can lead to markedly reduced sperm counts," notes Dr. Feinberg.

YOUR IDEAL WEIGHT

Regular, moderate exercise is critical to keeping your body fat at its optimum fertility setting. Eating the right amount is also key.

"Women who are extraordinarily overweight or underweight stop ovulating," notes Ronald E. Burmeister, M.D., an infertility specialist with the Reproductive Health and Fertility Center in Rockford, Illinois, and assistant professor of obstetrics and gynecology at the University of Illinois College of Medicine at Rockford. "My theory is that nature has a lot of checks and balances. It's protecting these women from pregnancy because they have more complicated pregnancies, including premature delivery and birth defects."

In fact, about one in eight cases of primary infertility in women (the inability to conceive a first child) is the result of either obesity or too-low body weight. Even more surprising, nearly three-quarters of these women will conceive on their own if they correct their weight problem.

To find out if you and your partner weigh too much, too little, or just the right amount, you can each calculate your body mass index (BMI) by using the chart on page 84. BMI is highly correlated with total body fat and is calculated by dividing your body weight in pounds by your height in inches squared and then multiplying the result by 705. The final number applies to both men and women and indicates risk for a number of weight-related health problems, including infertility.

An ideal BMI falls in the 20 to 24 range and should be your target for peak fertility. (Some doctors now believe a better range is 20 to 27, but more studies are needed.) Tremendous variation exists within this ideal range. For instance, a 5-foot 3-inch woman who weighs 120 pounds is in the same league as a 6-foot 2-inch man who weighs 160 pounds. Both have a fertility-fostering BMI of 21.

A BMI below 20, and particularly below 17, puts you and your partner in the fertility-robbing underweight range. A BMI of 25 to 30 (especially above 27) thrusts you into the worrisome overweight range. And if your

BMI is above 30 (obese), you are at the greatest risk for infertility. (Bear in mind, however, that these ranges measure a proportionate risk; there is no magic threshold when it comes to BMI.)

YES, YOU CAN BE *TOO* THIN

A certain amount of body fat provides the essential nutrients to support a growing fetus. But long before you get pregnant, the right amount of body fat also bolsters fertility by metabolizing the estrogens and estrogen precursors needed for ovulation and prompting brain messages that regulate reproductive hormones.

Fat cells produce a protein called leptin, which acts as a hormone and communicates with the reproductive system. If a woman's leptin levels are low because she is too thin, her reproductive system will receive a "distress" signal.

In turn, she begins turning estradiol (the principal female hormone) into 2-hydroxyestrone—an antiestrogen. This estrogen deficiency eventually results in irregular, unpredictable periods, dwindling secretions of vaginal mucus, lost sex drive, and ultimately dysfunctional ovulation. Many women who are infertile or subfertile will begin to produce an egg, but it never leaves the ovary. In other cases, the egg may be released, but the signal from the pituitary gland to produce progesterone may be interrupted or inadequate. Women may not be aware that a problem exists because their menstrual cycles are generally regular.

The link between weight and fertility in men isn't as well understood, but guys who are too slender may have decreased sperm function and lower sperm counts as a result of inadequate production of their male sex hormones.

If you or your partner has a BMI below 20 and you're trying for a baby—or plan to in the future—consider adding enough additional pounds to put you in the optimum 20 to 24 range. Those few extra pounds might just make the difference.

(continued on page 86)

BODY MASS INDEX...

Use the following chart adapted from the American Society for Reproductive Medicine to calculate your body mass index (BMI), which measures your weight-related health risk and can predict whether your weight is putting you at risk for infertility. The chart is accurate for both men and women, so be sure to have

Height	Weight (lb)									
	110	120	130	140	150	160	170	180	190	200
4'10"	23	25	27	29	31	34	36	38	40	42
4'11"	22	24	26	28	30	32	34	36	38	40
5'0"	22	23	25	27	29	31	33	35	37	39
5'1"	21	23	25	27	28	30	32	34	36	38
5'2"	20	22	24	26	27	29	31	33	35	37
5'3"	20	21	23	25	27	28	30	32	34	36
5'4"	19	21	22	24	26	28	29	31	33	34
5'5"	18	20	22	23	25	27	28	30	32	33
5'6"	18	19	21	23	24	26	27	29	31	32
5'7"	17	19	20	22	24	25	27	28	30	31
5'8"	17	18	20	21	23	24	26	27	29	30
5'9"	16	18	19	21	22	24	25	27	28	30
5'10"	16	17	19	20	22	23	24	26	27	29
5'11"	15	17	18	20	21	22	24	25	27	28
6'0"	15	16	18	19	20	22	23	24	26	27
6'1"	15	16	17	19	20	21	22	24	25	26
6'2"	14	15	17	18	19	21	22	23	24	26

...AND FERTILITY

Now that you've calculated your BMI, use the following chart to evaluate how this measurement may be impacting your conception odds. Though the link between body fat and fertility isn't as clear for men, those who drop below a BMI of 18 may begin to experience decreased libido and sperm defects. Thus, your partner may want to keep his BMI in the "peak fertility" range, too.

your partner check it out as well. To calculate your BMI, simply find your weight in the top column, then follow that column down until you hit the row for your height. The number at the intersection is your BMI.

Once you've determined your BMI, consult the second chart, which will help you to evaluate the effect on fertility your body mass index might have.

210	220	230	240	250	260	270	280	290	300	310	320
44	46	48	50	52	54	57	59	61	63	65	67
43	45	47	49	51	53	55	57	59	61	63	65
41	43	45	47	49	51	53	55	57	59	61	63
40	42	44	45	47	49	51	53	55	57	59	61
38	40	42	44	46	48	49	51	53	55	57	59
37	39	41	43	44	46	48	50	51	53	55	57
36	38	40	41	43	45	46	48	50	52	53	55
35	37	38	40	42	43	45	47	48	50	52	53
34	36	37	39	40	42	44	45	47	49	50	52
33	35	36	38	39	41	42	44	46	47	49	50
32	34	35	37	38	40	41	43	44	46	47	49
31	33	34	36	37	38	40	41	43	44	46	47
30	32	33	35	36	37	39	40	42	43	45	46
29	31	32	34	35	36	38	39	41	42	43	45
29	30	31	33	34	35	37	38	39	41	42	43
28	29	30	32	33	34	36	37	38	40	41	42
27	28	30	31	32	33	35	36	37	39	40	41

BMI	Effect on Female Fertility
Under 17	High risk of infertility
17 to 19	Slight risk of infertility
20 to 24	Peak fertility
25 to 27	No significant increase in infertility risk
28 to 30	Slight risk of infertility
Over 30	High risk of infertility

Of course, the thought of *adding* pounds to become healthier might seem counterintuitive in our weight-obsessed culture, where thin is most definitely in. Society tells us—and many women believe—that the more we diet and exercise, the healthier and more attractive we are. Admitting that your small dress size could be robbing you of full fertility is hard, and rounding out those ultra-svelte body lines with extra pounds may be even harder.

Doctors advise taking it slow—gaining one-half pound a week. Often 6 months is enough to restore reproductive function and get pregnant. Talk to your doctor or a nutritionist about a weight-gain plan that's right for you.

Finally, "many patients with a low BMI have psychological eating problems, like bulimia or anorexia nervosa," Dr. Burmeister notes. If this is true for you, seek out psychological help to resolve your eating disorder so that you can be at your healthiest when you begin trying to conceive.

BIGGER IS NOT BETTER

"The majority of overweight patients I see are just consuming too much of a good old-fashioned American diet, which is high in fat," notes Dr. Burmeister. But according to reproductive endocrinologist and gynecologic surgeon Deborah Metzger, M.D., Ph.D., medical director of Helena Women's Health in San Jose, California, and medical advisor to this book, the real culprit may be overindulging in carbohydrates. A carb-loaded diet creates ovulation chaos when excessive insulin and androgens (male hormones) build up in the blood.

The impact can be deadly to fertility. Like thin women, obese women often stop ovulating, but by a completely different process. Instead of converting estradiol to antiestrogens, their bodies turn up estrogen production. But what they produce are weaker estrogens—estrone and estriol—which eventually halt ovulation. In a double whammy, these women's bodies also increase production of androgens, which may affect egg production directly. Men who weigh too much may experience diminished fertility, too, but the process isn't fully understood.

Not all obese women have fertility problems, but many will notice their menstrual cycles becoming irregular and longer—a sign of increased estrone and estriol production. Dark hairs may also appear on their lower abdomen, face, and between their breasts, indicating that their ovaries are producing more of the male hormones androstenedione and testosterone. The more a woman weighs, the more of these fertility-robbing hormones she's likely to produce.

The evidence against fat is overwhelming. In one study, women with a BMI higher than 27 were approximately three times more likely to be infertile than women in the normal BMI range. What's more, the more weight you carry when you're younger, the greater your risk of infertility later on. Having an over-30 BMI at age 18 more than doubles your later infertility risk.

Even overweight women undergoing assisted reproduction treatment face greater fertility hurdles. A recent study found that very obese women (those with a BMI greater than 35) were 60 percent less likely to conceive during infertility treatment than women with BMIs of 20 to 24.9.

"If you are overweight and are having menstrual irregularity, it's going to help to lose weight," notes Stephen G. Somkuti, M.D., Ph.D., director of the in vitro fertilization program at Abington Memorial Hospital in Pennsylvania and assistant clinical professor at Jefferson Medical College in Philadelphia. "You may not have to lose hundreds of pounds. Losing only a few pounds may increase your fertility a few percentage points." And those few percentage points could be all it takes to become pregnant.

In fact, if you are overweight, dropping just 5 to 10 percent of your body weight (10 to 20 pounds if you weigh 200) can dramatically improve ovulation and your ability to get pregnant. You'll also cut your risk of miscarriage, pregnancy-related diabetes, high blood pressure, and having a high-birth-weight baby.

SYNDROME O

A significant benefit of losing weight is that it cuts insulin overproduction—which lies at the heart of some weight-related female fertility problems, including polycystic ovary syndrome (PCOS), otherwise known as Stein–Leventhal disease. Dr. Feinberg dubs these problems syndrome O in his forthcoming book, *Giving Your Fertility a Fighting Chance When Syndrome O Challenges You*, and groups the condition with a larger cluster of insulin-related disorders—including obesity, type 2 diabetes, and heart disease—called syndrome X.

Syndrome O is characterized by overnourishment, ovarian confusion, and ovulation disruption. Eighty to 90 percent of women with syndrome O are overweight, or "overnourished," according to Dr. Feinberg. They eat too much, particularly carbohydrate-rich snack foods that contain partially hydrogenated oils or trans fats, and rarely exercise. Both contribute to insulin overproduction.

Insulin keeps the body running by continually shuttling blood sugar, or glucose, into cells. When this process is derailed, the body can become insulin-resistant—more and more insulin must be produced by the pancreas in order for cells to respond to insulin and acquire the glucose necessary for energy production. Fat cells, however, remain insulin-sensitive and readily take up and use glucose to make fat. When insulin-resistant, the body is tricked into believing that it needs more insulin to feed glucose-starved cells. It responds by stepping up insulin production, but because cells are still insulin-resistant, an excess of insulin and sometimes glucose begins building up. Extra glucose is converted to fat (meaning additional pounds), which, in turn, causes cells to become *more* insulin-resistant—and churn out more insulin. It's a vicious cycle with serious consequences for fertility.

Out-of-whack insulin levels can eventually cause ovarian confusion, in which the ovaries fail to produce key female hormones and overproduce male hormones, disrupting the tiny egg follicles and leading to polycystic ovaries and ovulation disruption. Many insulin-resistant women are actually *hypo*glycemic. Whether your insulin levels are increased or decreased, you can improve insulin sensitivity through a healthful diet, exercise, and weight loss. This is central to restoring fertility. For specific nutritional advice for blood sugar control and maintaining fertility-fostering insulin levels, review the tips in chapter 3.

Whether you have PCOS or are just overweight, starting on a weight-loss plan now by losing a pound a week will put you ahead of the fertility game—even if you're not yet ready to conceive. "Take 15 months or 2 years, whatever is needed, to regain your ideal weight," Dr. Burmeister advises. You'll need to eat more mindfully and stick with an exercise program. "It takes time and a whole change in lifestyle," he concedes. But the benefits will be well worth it.

6

The Stress Connection

Shortly before her marriage at age 32, Katie Boland visited her doctor to learn just how much damage an earlier chlamydia infection had inflicted on her reproductive system. Diagnosis: blocked fallopian tubes. Chance of conception: 20 percent.

After the wedding, Katie launched an all-out quest to find a fertility specialist who could help her get pregnant. Three frustrating years later, after consulting several doctors and undergoing numerous fertility treatments, including a laparoscopy to open her blocked tubes, she still hadn't conceived. But the most devastating news came when her doctor diagnosed her with lupus, a potentially fatal and incurable autoimmune disease.

"I was lost and insane," she recalls. "I kept wondering, how am I going to make this pregnancy happen? Finally I realized I just had to make myself well, stay open, and trust that my baby would come when she was ready."

At the suggestion of friends and her therapist, she began reading self-help books about how negative and stressful thoughts can lead to physical disorders, including lupus and infertility. Katie stopped her traditional fertility treatment, began exercising regularly, and changed her diet to include more fruits and vegetables, less fat, more whole grains, and no sugar. She also focused on reframing negative thoughts into positive ones, envisioning herself with a healthy body and baby.

"I did everything I could to calm myself down," she recalls, including doing breathing exercises to de-stress, indulging in quiet walks and leisurely baths, pampering herself at spas, and practicing prayer and meditation. She even achieved her dream of writing a screenplay. Three months later, her lupus went into remission, and 6 weeks after that—just shy of her 36th birthday—she discovered she was pregnant with her daughter Mimi.

"It's all about stress," Katie asserts. "I really believe it plays a role in infertility, just like it does with high blood pressure and heart problems. Addressing it in a meaningful way really makes a difference."

In addition to being a mom, Katie went on to detail her stress-busting strategies in a book, *I Got Pregnant, You Can Too! How Healing Yourself Physically, Mentally, and Spiritually Leads to Fertility.*

FIGHT OR FLIGHT

For centuries, healers intuitively sensed a link between infertility and stress—that is, until modern medicine arrived and pooh-poohed the notion that infertility is caused by anything other than physical maladies that can be seen and fixed. Stress, it was concluded, is all in the mind—not in the reproductive organs.

Even so, the idea that emotions and fertility are somehow connected never completely died away, partly because of stories like Katie Boland's. "People point to anecdotes, such as couples who adopt and then get pregnant," notes Scott J. Roseff, M.D., director of the West Essex Center for Advanced Reproductive Endocrinology in West Orange, New Jersey, and clinical associate professor in the obstetrics and gynecology department at the University of Medicine and Dentistry of New Jersey. "I can't tell you how many times that happens—over and over and over again. Or couples who go through aggressive means to get pregnant, have a baby, and suddenly they're pregnant again on their own. It's like now the pressure's off and there's no more stress."

Stress, it has since been discovered, isn't only in the mind. It's also a physical reaction, shaped by millions of years of evolution in an eat-or-be-eaten world—a physical reaction that touches nearly every system in the body, including reproduction.

For much of human history, this "fight-or-flight" response to stress served us well. When we were confronted with life-threatening situations, like a saber-toothed tiger or a mudslide, the brain's hypothalamus sounded a distress call, pumping stress hormones into our bodies to push up our heart rates and send a burst of energy to muscles to help us either flee or fight. Once we were safe, the hypothalamus signaled our bodies and minds to calm down. Famed Harvard cardiologist Herbert Benson, M.D., dubbed this the "relaxation response" back in the 1960s.

"In our current society, though, we have the fight-or-flight response virtually every day as a result of job stress, long commutes, and so on. That's not normal," says reproductive endocrinologist and gynecologic surgeon Deborah Metzger, M.D., Ph.D., medical director of Helena Women's Health in San Jose, California, and medical advisor to this book.

Chronic stress keeps our minds and bodies in a perpetual state of high alert, like a firefighter forced, day after day, to answer repeated false alarms. Our health eventually suffers, resulting in depression, immune system disorders, and other physical and mental breakdowns. And because the hypothalamus also coordinates the body's hormonal and nervous systems, including the secretion of reproductive hormones from the nearby pituitary gland, ovulation and sperm production are often disrupted, too.

Indeed, stress-related hormonal imbalances have been shown to scramble or stop menstrual cycles and cause fallopian tubes to spasm, barricading eggs from entering the uterus, says Alice Domar, Ph.D., founder and director of the Mind/Body Program for Infertility at Boston IVF, an infertility clinic affiliated with Beth Israel Deaconess Medical Center and Harvard Medical School. High stress is also linked to abnormal or lower sperm production and impotence in men.

STRESS BY ANY OTHER NAME

One of the most significant recent findings is that not all types of stress threaten fertility equally. In other words, it isn't necessarily the stress, say, of pursuing a high-intensity—but enjoyable—career or getting the jitters before a big presentation that causes reproductive woes. Rather, it's your long-term emotional reaction to traumatic or uncontrollable life events. That includes the devastation of an infertility diagnosis, which may compound an already existing inability to conceive.

"Until the 1990s, researchers had always viewed the stress of infertility as *anxiety* about not getting pregnant (accompanied by racing thoughts, edginess, tense muscles, and sweaty palms)," notes Dr. Domar, coauthor of *Six Steps to Increased Fertility* and author of *Conquering Infertility*. Yet researchers were unable to prove a direct link between anxiety and the rate of conception. "But if you define stress as *depression* or *psychological distress* (characterized by feelings of hopelessness, sadness, pessimism, lack of interest in things once enjoyed, and changes in appetite), then it seems to have an impact on the conception rate," she notes.

Indeed, women with a history of depression experience infertility twice as often as other women, and those who are most depressed at the outset of in vitro fertilization (IVF) are significantly less likely to get pregnant than women who aren't depressed. In one study, for instance, depressed women who had already undergone several IVF cycles had a 13 percent pregnancy rate, compared to the 29 percent pregnancy rate of women who weren't depressed before IVF treatment.

Perhaps the strongest evidence that distress and depression hamper conception comes from studies showing that receiving psychological treatment boosts fertility. In one of the most conclusive studies ever done, Dr. Domar and her colleagues found that women who'd been trying to conceive for 1 to 2 years were significantly more likely to get pregnant after participating in either a 10-week cognitive-behavioral program similar to the one Dr. Domar now offers, including stress management strategies, relaxation training, and nutritional and exercise advice, or in 10 sessions of a support group focusing on different aspects of infertility, including self-esteem, marriage, and job. After one year, 55 percent of the cognitive-behavioral program participants and 54 percent of the support-group participants had given birth, compared to only 20 percent of control group participants, who received standard fertility treatment.

The message is clear: Negative emotions and psychological stress needn't rule your reproductive life. Mental strain can be tamed and overcome. So, even if you and your partner are still years away from pregnancy, finding time to calm down and cultivate serenity is sure to keep your reproductive engines in optimum working order for later on. And if you've been trying to conceive for a while, learning to rein in noxious emotions could give your mind and body just the fertility boost needed to conceive.

"Stress interferes with the ability to get pregnant, but it's not an absolute," notes Dr. Metzger. "The only absolute is if your tubes are blocked or you don't have sperm. My approach is to decrease some of the factors that contribute to infertility—and stress is one."

ARE YOU STRESSED OUT?

It's all too easy to continue functioning under chronic stress, brushing aside worries and weariness and ignoring your body's subtle pleas to heed a gentler internal rhythm. Even the havoc wreaked on your reproductive hormones may be too subtle to change your menstrual cycles or your partner's sperm counts—at least at first. "Then one day, your body suddenly can't compensate anymore and it crashes," Dr. Metzger explains. For many, stress-related illnesses, infertility, and mental exhaustion come as a complete surprise.

"You may not realize that you're stressed," Dr. Metzger says. "One way to tell is if something comes up unexpectedly and it totally overwhelms you. Or every minute of your day is scheduled. The key is making time that's not planned. It's okay to have part of the day when you're not doing something. In fact, it's incredibly healthy."

Finding ways to foster tranquility in your life should keep stress at bay and boost your lifelong reproductive health. Even the most dedicated serenity-seekers, however, occasionally fall prey to calm-crushing life circumstances. If stress or negative feelings ever threaten to overwhelm you or persist for more than a few days, consider seeking help from friends and family or a professional. According to the American Society for Reproductive Medicine, warning signs include:

* Loss of interest in usual activities

* Depression that doesn't lift

* Strained interpersonal relationships (with your partner, family, friends, or colleagues)

* High levels of anxiety

* A diminished ability to accomplish tasks

* Difficulty concentrating

* Change in your sleep patterns (trouble falling asleep or staying asleep, early-morning awakening, or sleeping more than usual)

* Changes in appetite or weight (increase or decrease)

* Increased alcohol or drug use

* Thoughts about death or suicide

* Social isolation

* Persistent feelings of pessimism, guilt, or worthlessness

* Chronic feelings of bitterness or anger

DE-STRESS AT HOME

The earlier you and your partner learn to defuse mental stress and negative emotions, the better your long-term health will be and the greater your reproductive odds when the time comes to conceive. If you're already trying to get pregnant, daily stress-busting could speed up your time to conception.

Dr. Domar recommends practicing some form of relaxation every day for 20 minutes. Whether you choose to do breathing exercises, guided imagery, yoga, or some other technique, the idea is to elicit the relaxation response to slow your heart rate, breathing, and brain waves to below normal resting levels.

Here are a few simple do-it-yourself exercises, drawn from Dr. Domar's 10-week Mind/Body Program for Infertility. Both you and your partner can try these at home to decrease stress and optimize fertility, no matter where you are in your reproductive journey.

Don't feel guilty if you can't find time every day to do your relaxation exercise. Just keep coming back to it. Eventually, it will be such a rewarding part of your life, you won't want to miss a day.

Use imagery to create calm. Guided imagery is one of the most powerful tools for cultivating tranquility, says Dr. Domar. Use an audiotape to guide you or develop your own imagery. Here's an exercise to try.

1. Sit comfortably in a quiet place.

2. Take several slow, deep breaths.

3. Picture in your mind's eye a place that you love or have felt relaxed in.

4. Visualize yourself strolling or sitting or standing there, slowly taking in the views, sounds, and fragrances.

5. If the place is outdoors, view the color of the sky, the shape of the clouds, the greens of the grass and leaves, and the ocean waves—whatever surrounds you.

6. Concentrate on the smells: sun-warmed grass, moist leaves, salty air, rainwater freshness.

7. Focus on the sounds: squirrels chattering, bird songs, music, rain falling on the roof.

8. Explore the sensations you feel—the sun's warmth on your face, the tickle of grass between your toes, damp sand under your bare feet.

9. Allow yourself to sink into these sensations and relish your pleasure and comfort. Take note of anxious thoughts for a moment, then return to the sights, sounds, and sensations around you.

Don't worry if it's difficult at first to transport yourself to an imaginary place. To help, try imagining yourself being whisked there on a magic carpet or envision yourself floating there on your own, as if you were flying.

Take a mini-relaxation break with deep breathing. Besides your regular relaxation practice, you may want to include some shorter breathing exercises for times when you're feeling upset or anxious, such as right before that big job performance review or while you're stuck in traffic. The goal is to shift from quick, shallow breathing—which allows only a limited amount of oxygen to reach our brains and bodies—to deep, calming abdominal breathing. These exercises can be done in public without others even knowing.

Here are two from Dr. Domar.

1. Sit or lie down in a comfortable position.

2. Take a deep, slow breath, directing your breathing into your abdomen. It sometimes helps to breathe in with your nose and out through your mouth.

3. Place a hand on your abdomen. Keep your stomach muscles relaxed, and allow your abdomen to rise about an inch as you inhale. Notice that your chest also rises slightly with your abdomen.

4. As you exhale, your abdomen will fall about an inch. Your diaphragm (the partition separating your chest and abdominal cavities) should move down as you inhale and up as you exhale. If your diaphragm isn't moving, you're not breathing abdominally.

Or try this:

1. While concentrating on breathing from your abdomen rather than your chest, count down from 10 to zero, taking one complete breath—one inhale and one exhale—with each number (10 for the first inhale and exhale, 9 for the second, and so on).

2. By the time you reach zero, you should feel more relaxed. If not, try again.

Nurture yourself. Women have a particularly tough time ministering to their own needs and building pleasure into their lives. Many see their role as nurturer to everyone but themselves. If you have a tendency to put yourself last, it's time to rethink your nurturing strategy and count yourself among those you cherish.

Think about the hobbies and activities that bring you joy and write them down. They can be simple things, like soaking in a tub with aro-

FERTILITY VISIONARIES

Alice Domar, Ph.D., and the Mind/Body Program for Infertility

While she was completing her graduate training at Beth Israel Deaconess Medical Center in Boston, Alice Domar, Ph.D., and her colleagues had a sudden "aha" experience. Having studied with Harvard's Herbert Benson, M.D., who discovered the body's "relaxation response," Dr. Domar was familiar with the hypothalamus's role in gearing up the body to either fight or flee in response to stress, then calm down again once the danger passed. She also knew it had a hand in regulating reproductive hormones. Could it be, she and the others wondered, that ongoing stress—living in a perpetual state of fight-or-flight—hurts fertility? And, if so, might eliciting the relaxation response counteract the harm?

To test their hunch, they designed a study of 100 infertile women. Half would learn techniques designed to induce the relaxation response along with tradtional medical treatment for infertility, and the other half would receive only traditional treatment. When women who were receiving only medical treatment started showing up in tears, despondent over their inability to conceive, however, Dr. Domar decided to forgo the study as envisioned and teach them all relaxation techniques.

"That was 1987," she says, referring to the birth of her pioneering Mind/Body Program for Infertility. "Thousands of patients later, my office is covered with baby pictures." About 44 percent of Dr. Domar's patients become pregnant within 6 months—even those who've been trying for up to 10 years.

Far more meaningful, though, are the psychological gains made by participants, notes Dr. Domar. About 95 percent see their lives turned around emotionally and spiritually—whether or not they eventually conceive. "I really

matherapy oils, going on a hike, getting a manicure, reading a good novel, taking a nap, sitting by a fire, or just spending time with people who nurture and support you.

Draw a circle and divide it into pie slices of varying sizes to represent the activities you do during a typical day and how long you spend doing them. Try cutting down on the activities that zap your spirit and add more of the pastimes you relish. With a little forethought, for instance, you can

started the program to help women cope with infertility," she explains. "They come in entirely miserable—they've hit bottom. When they leave 10 weeks later, it's amazing how much better they are. I consider pregnancy a nice bonus."

Dr. Domar has since moved an expanded version of her program to Boston IVF, an infertility clinic affiliated with Beth Israel Deaconess Medical Center and Harvard Medical School. Patients enrolled in the program participate in 10 sessions, each focusing on different coping techniques. These include guided imagery, mini-relaxation breathing techniques, yoga, mindfulness, and cognitive restructuring (eliminating corrosive thoughts and replacing them with positive affirmations). Participants also learn how to focus on nurturing themselves, express painful emotions through journaling, and say no to requests that don't serve their emotional or physical health. The groups are mostly for women, though partners participate in 3 of the 10 sessions. The activities in these shared sessions include paired listening exercises, which are designed to help couples work through problems in their relationship related to infertility.

Contact information: To participate in Dr. Domar's program or learn about other infertility programs at Boston IVF, log on to www.bostonivf.com, e-mail her at conqueringinfertility@bostonivf.com, or call (781) 434-6500. Dr. Domar also offers 1-hour telephone consultations from anywhere in the world and runs shorter weekend retreats around the United States based on her 10-week course. For names of affiliate mind–body infertility programs nationwide, check the Mind/Body Medical Institute's Web site at www.mbmi.org. Dr. Domar is also the author of the book *Conquering Fertility*.

learn to combine multiple trips to the grocery store into one, leaving extra hours to pursue what fulfills you.

Practice mindfulness. You may be so fixated on earning a promotion at work or reliving every word of the spat you had last night with your partner that you forget to focus on what's happening here and now. By being mindful of this particular moment, you start to slow down and savor the task at hand—whether it's washing vegetables or making love. The world around you and your body's sensations become more vibrant and stress melts away.

Here's a mindfulness exercise from Dr. Domar.

1. Pick up an orange, noticing its skin texture and the way it smells.

2. Peel it slowly, piece by piece, focusing on the citrus fragrance.

3. Gently tear each segment apart, noticing the symmetry between segments.

4. As you bite into each piece, concentrate on the ooze of juice and the tang of citrus in your nose and mouth.

5. Savor every taste, including the last bit of juice that you lick from your fingers.

If you notice your mind wandering or other thoughts intruding as you practice this exercise, don't chastise yourself or fight it. Recognize that thoughts move in and out of consciousness all the time. Simply observe them and return your attention to whatever you're doing.

Give voice to painful emotions. Career demands, difficult relationships, painful episodes from the past—all of these things can make you anxious or angry, robbing you of full reproductive health. Learning to regularly voice anger or other painful emotions—even if you can't directly confront those you're angry with—is one of the healthiest things you can do for your long-term stress management and fertility.

Keep a journal and write down everything you feel and why—not just angry feelings, but any grief, worry, sorrow, or frustrations you may be carrying inside, including emotions buried from the past. Printing it out in black and white will help you recognize and reconcile distressing emotions you maybe didn't even know were there. With time and soul-searching, you should gain real insights into your emotional makeup and learn to halt harmful feelings before they take root. (To learn more about how journaling can be used to prepare for future parenthood, see chapter 7.)

Listen to each other. Even if you and your partner are still years away from starting a family, learning to listen to each other—really listen—will strengthen your bond and make you better parents when the time comes. After all, the time to work on a ruptured relationship isn't after you've conceived, but well before. And if you're currently trying to get pregnant, regular communication will help you and your partner head off any fertility frustrations that may arise *before* they cause cracks in your relationship.

Sit with your partner, taking turns talking while the other listens. Dr. Domar recommends discussing three topics: something you like about your partner that you've never mentioned; something you like about yourself that you've never revealed; and some unspoken thing you like about your relationship. Then let your partner have a turn. (We'll discuss additional relationship-strengthening strategies in chapters 7 and 13.)

Empower yourself to say no. Women especially have a hard time saying no to requests for their time and emotional energy, often at the expense of their health. Have your partner or a friend read a list of requests that are hard to turn down ("Can I borrow a quarter for a phone call? Will you come over for dinner?"). Dr. Domar advises saying no in three different ways: a simple no; no, but how about such and such; and no, because . . . and give a good reason for turning down the request. The key is learning to set boundaries and cultivate peace of mind.

7

Finding Inner Order

Just as good nutrition is important when you are planning a pregnancy, spiritual and psychological nourishment are essential, too. The more you contribute to your personal growth in all the years leading up to conception, the better prepared your mind and body will be for the experience of becoming a parent.

"Long before you pour yourself into gestating a baby, your job is to grow your own self into wholeness," explains Deborah Issokson, Psy.D., a psychologist specializing in counseling for reproductive health and healing and a faculty member of both the Massachusetts School of Professional Psychology in Boston and Boston University's Nurse-Midwifery Education Program.

It takes soul-searching to know and fulfill your deepest needs as a conscious adult, while perceiving your future child's needs, says Carista Luminare-Rosen, Ph.D., a California-based counselor who specializes in holistic approaches to preconception and prenatal health and is the author of *Parenting Begins before Conception*.

"A true holistic approach to preconception preparation involves the recognition that a mom, a dad, and a child each have four bodies that need to be taken care of with equal concern," Dr. Luminare-Rosen explains. "In addition to a strong *physical body*, a healthy *emotional body* can express the full range of experiences, from the darker feelings to the more buoyant feelings. A healthy *mental body* puts forth thoughts and attitudes that benefit your own well-being, your relationships, your community, and, ultimately, a future child. *Spiritual health* is a wellspring of positive ideals, values, and beliefs."

By attending to unhealed wounds and recognizing any imbalances in these four bodies, you can move closer to nourishing all aspects of the self. Then, your most loving nature and inner wisdom will resonate as you conceive and become parents.

SET PREPARENTING PRIORITIES

As you open your heart to the concept of having a child, remember *all* of the roles you are preparing for. "In addition to being effective in your career, you'll find yourself trying to remain true to yourself, while being a reliable source of love for your family, a beloved to your partner, and a friend to your community," points out Dr. Luminare-Rosen. Your self-esteem and self-expression may need some attention in order to optimize these roles. "I also recommend that you take careful inventory of how you allocate your time and energy," she says. Most likely, certain responsibilities and aspirations will need to shift to meet the demands of parenting.

"If the idea of sacrifice is difficult for you or your partner, embrace the idea that having a baby is a profound spiritual journey," says Dr. Luminare-Rosen. "Not only does your baby need you, but you need your baby to develop yourself. You are not only conceiving a child but recreating and rebirthing yourself as you expand your consciousness for the miraculous events that will occur within you and your partner."

Here are some guidelines to start making room for future parenthood in your life.

Evaluate your career path. If your plan is to concentrate on your career now and get pregnant after you've established yourself professionally, be

WHAT WORKED FOR US
LYNNE AND MICHAEL CAME "HOME" TO START THEIR FAMILY

Lynne Eshleman Brolly always heard adults remark how the rural Pennsylvania town where she grew up was ideal for raising a family. Admittedly, she had had a happy childhood in the world of farmers' markets, folk festivals, and 4-H clubs. But as a small-college-town girl with big dreams, she made a break for New York City when she came of age.

In the city, she became a successful wood finisher and developed her passions for yoga, meditation, and vegetarian cooking. But no matter where she went, her roots still remained strong. Michael, the man Lynne married, actually went to college in her hometown and had the same livelihood as her grandfather, a woodworker. The horse-and-buggy–traveled roads of her hometown often lured Lynne back to visit her sisters, father, stepmother, and growing number of nieces and nephews.

After New York, Lynne and Michael moved to an artist colony in Virginia. It was there that the couple decided to start trying for a baby. At the time, Lynne was 36 and Michael was 49. It wasn't until career opportunities brought the couple back to Lynne's hometown, though, that baby Hugh was actually conceived. "I don't think it's any coincidence that it was when we finally decided to 'settle down'—especially among friends and family—that I got pregnant," Lynne comments.

They purchased their first house (a fixer-upper farmhouse), bought their first new car, joined a lively church in the heart of town, Lynne started a new job, and they found out Lynne was pregnant, all in 1 month. "It was like I grew up all at once. After coming back on my terms, I was able to embrace the community that I maybe took a little for granted before," says Lynne.

Just 10 months after Hugh was born, the couple conceived their second child, Liam. (By this time, Lynne was 38 and Michael was 51.)

Lynne attributes her easy conceptions and great childbirth experiences to being truly at home—comfortable within her body, secure in her marriage, balanced in her lifestyle, and supported by her community.

sure your work *contributes to* and doesn't *deplete* your vital energy, emphasizes Dr. Luminare-Rosen. The best measure of the sustainability of your job is your exhaustion level, she says. "Work, by its very nature, can make you tired, but the wrong work will leave you feeling burnt out and out of balance. I find that when women are in a career where they truly follow their hearts, they aren't as likely to drive themselves in unhealthy ways."

"Of course, even women with heart-loving careers and vocations can still run themselves ragged," she points out. "What is most essential is to rebalance and nurture yourself when you feel depleted or empty after a day of work." (Review the advice in chapter 6 for specific relaxation and renewal guidelines.)

Allow yourself to grieve your child-free life. The word *grief* never shows up in pregnancy literature, so women think they're not supposed to associate grief with welcoming a baby into their lives. But even in the most wanted, planned situations, people are somewhat bittersweet about altering their lifestyles and relationships, says Dr. Issokson. "It's okay to talk about how you might be ecstatic about having a baby, but yet you're really going to miss carefree get-togethers with friends, romantic mornings with your partner, your disposable income, and the like. There are so many levels of loss with a life change as profound as parenthood. Loss brings grief. Give yourself permission to acknowledge both your anticipated joy *and* anticipated sadness and all the ambivalence in between," she says.

Keep a journal. Your evolving consciousness of future parenthood can be supported by keeping a journal, notes Dr. Luminare-Rosen. "Consider beginning your journal by examining your fear as well as your excitement about becoming a parent. Let your journal be your confidante, and be truthful about your innermost desires and concerns," she says. Daily writing can help you manage relationship issues, career challenges, and wounds from your childhood. At the same time, you may be inspired to reach out to your unborn child through letters, pictures, and poems. Any connection you open up now will foster a greater bond in the future.

Prepare physical space. Physically assessing the space you need for a baby's clothes, furniture, and toys can help you mentally make space for a baby in your life. "Now is the time to consider if your living space can guarantee the room, safety, and security needed for a baby," says Dr. Luminare-Rosen. Since moving or renovating is a long and arduous process, it's ideal to start before you're pregnant, she points out.

Revisit your finances. Take inventory of your income and expenses, including investments, personal belongings, vacations, and costs ofdaily living. Now consider what needs to shift to also include maternity leave, child care, medical care, and living arrangements for a child. Discuss with your partner what each of you is and isn't willing to give up to create a spending plan that takes care of everyone's needs, advises Dr. Luminare-Rosen.

Fulfill your dreams. Be honest. If you have a burning desire to explore the Australian outback, finish your novel, or complete your degree, it's not going to be easy during pregnancy or early parenthood. If unfulfilled dreams might prevent opening your heart to parenting, get on the fast track to fulfilling them by imposing a deadline. But be selective. Many of your ambitions will need to be relinquished or put on hold with the realization that parenting demands compromise and sacrifice for a greater good, Dr. Luminare-Rosen says.

READY YOUR RELATIONSHIP

Co-parenting will allow you and your partner to become more selfless, loving, patient, and persevering. You can use all of the challenges of parenthood to attain a spiritual depth that brings out the best in you as individuals and as a couple, says Dr. Luminare-Rosen.

Parenting is a journey that requires you to express your feelings and thoughts to one another with great finesse. "Differences are fine, if the couple can respect and embrace those differences and find common ground," Dr. Luminare-Rosen says. But expect relationship vulnerabilities to be exposed by the demands of co-parenting.

"Often, people have a fantasy that a baby will make the relationship better. If you are having relationship problems, babies won't solve them—babies create more complications and more stress," cautions Dr. Issokson.

A study involving more than 1,300 children and their parents noted that a woman locked in a stormy marriage runs more than double the risk of bearing a psychologically or physically damaged child than a woman in a secure, nurturing relationship.

The following advice will help you determine the strengths and weaknesses of your relationship and how to grow together as future parents.

Evaluate your communication dynamic. Does it feel like you and your partner are speaking different languages that leave you perplexed and frustrated? Do you bicker in a way that would be unhealthy for a future child to hear? "If your words or attitude disempower or devalue one another, you should seek couples counseling," says Dr. Luminare-Rosen. Numerous counseling techniques can teach you communications skills.

Establish bonds with children and families. While you're still thinking of starting a family, it's good practice for you and your partner to baby-sit together or do some volunteer work with children. These experiences are likely to bring out parenting concerns that still need attention, as well as experiences you look forward to. Also, spend time with families you know and ask them all you can about their parenting styles, so you can start to get a sense of what works for you.

Define roles and responsibilities. You and your partner may have different ideas about what a mother or father's role is, based on your unique upbringings and attitudes. It's never too early to clarify co-parenting expectations with one another, says Dr. Luminare-Rosen. Since you may need time to get on the same page, start sorting out your views on discipline and how you could work out your division of labor. Discuss things like who would drive the baby to day care, get up in the middle of the night, and keep up with household chores like grocery shopping, she advises.

Build your confidence. Even as you assess areas that need improvement, you and your partner should welcome the excitement and inspiration that comes with realizing what you have to offer. Tell your partner what talents and personality traits he has that will enrich your progeny. Mention anything from reliability and sense of humor to an appreciation for culture or athletics. Solicit a list of your assets from your partner, too, if he doesn't offer. Also, acknowledge the ways that you and you and your partner *together* can complement one another as co-parents.

Consider your "family values." "Explore how you and your partner hope to have a child within the larger context of the world. You may want to begin discussing how your environmental concerns, political viewpoints, religious alignments, educational standards, and moral principles will shape your vision of parenting," suggests Dr. Luminare-Rosen. "This is a great time to expose any potential conflicts as well as affirm perspectives that are compatible. Your parenting journey will continue to reveal op-

FERTILITYVISIONARIES

Niravi Payne, M.S., and The Whole Person Fertility Program

For decades, psychologists have been using a tool called a genogram to study family relationships. In 1983, psychotherapist Niravi B. Payne, M.S., developed the ephistogram, an emotional and physical family health history based on the principles of the genogram. The ephistogram formed the basis for the development of The Whole Person Fertility Program.

Whether used on its own or with medical fertility treatments, this program offers a broader view of fertility and is intended to heal the split between emotions and bodily responses. It has been responsible for assisting thousands of women and men in their efforts to conceive.

Payne's system maps out a person's in utero, birthing, and early childhood experiences in conjunction with the family's beliefs, thoughts, and patterns of behavior that affect the psyche and reproductive capacity. For example, a woman may have subconsciously picked up on her parents' reluctance about having her, or heard them say she was a "mistake." Memories like this may reemerge as hidden ambivalence or lack of confidence when a woman attempts to conceive. "Our endocrine, immune, and nervous systems are all intimately connected and influenced by every thought we think and every emotion we feel, which often throws off the delicately balanced hormonal system involved in reproduction and spermatogenesis," she explains.

In addition, Payne considers the unique social, political, and generational factors that play a role in a woman's fertility. "Many baby-boomer women emotionally disconnected from their mothers in the process of trying to set their generation apart from more traditional roles. Having tasted the liberating benefits of societal changes, many women expressed fears about a loss of

portunities to evaluate what values, beliefs, and attitudes you want to consciously pass on to your child."

HEAL UNHEALTHY PATTERNS

"If you are in an abusive or potentially abusive situation, don't by any means assume that getting pregnant will make things better," cautions Lisa

autonomy and financial independence should they have a child. When a woman feels ready to conceive, however, she is often unaware that her conflicts concerning childbearing have not been resolved," Payne notes.

"Your relationship with your father also affects how you view your body, embrace your sexuality, and relate to your mate—all issues that are crucial to conception and carrying a pregnancy to term," Payne explains. In addition, "the bonds we forge with our siblings are so primal and enduring that they shape our reproductive experiences more than we realize." Payne also considers the lives of grandparents and other relatives to identify any prevalent familial patterns, such as high divorce rates, substance abuse, and miscarriages.

To help a woman gain greater reproductive freedom, Payne will have the woman and her partner engage in activities such as writing about their lives, guided imagery, family photoanalysis, dream work, breathing exercises, and biofeedback. She'll also recommend lifestyle changes that have proven successful over her program's 20-year history.

Contact information: Call The Whole Person Fertility Program at (800) 666-HEAL or (239) 472-4092, or log on to www.niravi.com.

Counseling is done in person or over the phone. (You might also be able to encounter Payne at one of the many conferences and workshops she organizes or visits throughout the world.) In addition to exploring your ephistogram, Payne will provide counseling that revolves around an extensive Mind/Body Health, Attitudinal, and Lifestyle Profile, which also defines your current and past issues regarding family and conception.

Summers, C.N.M., Dr.P.H., a public health expert and spokesperson for the American College of Nurse-Midwives in Washington, D.C. Pregnancy is actually a time when physical abuse often begins or escalates. In addition to the long-term emotional damage to the mother, immediate concerns include miscarriage, hemorrhage, preterm labor, and rupture of the uterus.

If you have the slightest concerns for your safety, don't hesitate to talk to a doctor or nurse. "Battered women and their perpetrators come from all racial, ethnic, and religious groups, all socioeconomic levels, and all trades and professions. There's no shame in admitting that you need help," says Dr. Summers. Your doctor or nurse can connect you with social workers, legal aid, and counselors. You can also turn to your local social services department; the number is listed in your telephone book.

Likewise, pregnancy planning requires you to take urgent action on any *self-inflicted* abuse. Substance addiction, eating disorders, and dysfunctional relationships take time to resolve—experts recommend you stay on birth control until these patterns are well under control. When it comes to past abuse, it's in your future child's best interest to deal with unhealed emotional wounds. Having a child can evoke painful memories within you of your own history of childhood neglect, abuse, and unmet needs.

"Everyone has childhood wounds; they are inherent in growing up. The ones to be most concerned with are those that have left you with a sense that you can't provide your child with safe, healthy, and loving conditions 24 hours a day, 7 days a week," says Dr. Luminare-Rosen. "It's not like you have to have it all together before becoming pregnant. But if you are conscious of unhealthy patterns and committed to getting help when you need it, the chances that your child will inherit your wounds are greatly diminished," she says. "Anyone can learn to cultivate new aspects of their personality and reclaim undeveloped parts of themselves that were not nurtured during childhood. It doesn't mean that you won't have the painful memory, but you don't have to be run by the past if you choose to make the effort to become more self-aware of its detrimental effect on you. It is also a wonderful time to acknowledge the positive impact of your childhood experiences in your preparation for parenthood."

Consider the following advice, which is geared toward healing on all levels.

Check in with a therapist. Regardless of how happy or tragic your childhood may have been, Dr. Issokson encourages every potential parent to seek out at least one therapy session. "Because it is such a huge developmental time, preconception is an appropriate time to seek out counseling and support," she says. "If nothing else, a therapy session or meeting with a group can help you realize that your fears and concerns are normal. Women tend to think that their feelings are shameful or unusual just because they have never heard someone talk about these ideas."

Ease perfectionism. Despite the benefits of a great education and devoted parents, "advantaged women" can sometimes have such a drive to please that they have forgotten how to take care of themselves. "If you endured obsessively high standards in your upbringing, your work is to develop more compassion for yourself as you learn to self-nurture your body, mind, and spirit in more balanced ways," says Dr. Luminare-Rosen. "As an adult, you are free to define what is healthy for your well-being at any given moment."

Be honest about depression and anxiety. Statistically, women with clinical depression or anxiety are twice as likely as women without a mental health condition to experience fertility challenges. If you suspect a mental health disorder, get the help you need so your hormones and psyche are back in order by the time you want to conceive. (For a list of telltale symptoms, refer to page 95.)

Let nature connect you to your creative, nurturing self. The beauty and rhythm of the natural world can calm your nervous system and get you in sync with the balance and order of the universe. "As you get closer to conception, staying connected to the earth is so appropriate, since creating new life in the body *is* nature in its essence," says Dr. Issokson. She recommends that you bask in the natural world by gardening, caring for animals, swimming in the ocean, bird-watching, walking barefoot—whatever helps you feel nurtured and nurturing.

8

Contraception Savvy

Hormone-releasing IUDs. Depo-Provera. Vaginal rings. Fertility awareness methods. Determining your best contraceptive option is no easy feat—particularly if you want to prevent pregnancy now while also safeguarding your future fertility.

As you and your partner plumb the possibilities, think first about a contraceptive's ability to stave off sexually transmitted diseases (STDs), like gonorrhea, chlamydia, and syphilis, and its effectiveness against unwanted pregnancies. STDs, which often lead to pelvic inflammatory disease (PID), are a key cause of impaired fertility. And if your contraception fails and you become pregnant, complications such as miscarriage or a cesarean section could harm your future fertility.

"Other fertility-specific risks of various contraceptives are trivial to these," notes Felicia H. Stewart, M.D., adjunct professor of obstetrics and gynecology at the University of California, San Francisco, and codirector of the university's Center for Reproductive Health Research and Policy. (For more about STDs and other illnesses and medical treatments that harm fertility, see chapter 10.)

That's not to say, though, that contraceptives don't have a temporary impact on your ability to get pregnant after you stop using them. With some, you can conceive right away. With others, though, pregnancy may take months. If you're older, you may not have the luxury of time.

Here's a rundown of your contraceptive choices—the tried-and-true as well as some new arrivals—and their fertility-specific benefits and risks.

ORAL CONTRACEPTIVES

The Pill. Most popular is the "combined" Pill, which thickens the cervical mucus, making it less permeable to sperm, and makes the uterine lining unreceptive to an implanting embryo. It also releases synthetic estrogen and progestin into your system and jumbles the communication lines between your pituitary gland and ovaries to block ovulation. Normally, the pituitary gland coordinates the release of follicle-stimulating hormone (FSH) and luteinizing hormone (LH), which regulate the monthly release of an egg. The Pill stops the signal that prompts production of FSH and LH—essentially tricking the body into believing it's pregnant—and halts the cycle.

Breastfeeding mothers and other women who are estrogen-sensitive may opt for progestin-only pills, also known as minipills. Because they contain less progestin than combined pills and no estrogen, they don't always thwart ovulation. They're nearly as effective in preventing pregnancy as the combined Pill, however, even when ovulation occurs, because they also thicken cervical mucus and actually alter its molecular structure, making it hostile to sperm.

Fertility benefits: Taken every day, combined pills and minipills are nearly 100 percent effective against pregnancy. They also defend against fertility-harming ectopic, or tubal, pregnancies, in which the baby develops outside the uterus, usually in a fallopian tube. Surgery to remove the fetus and sometimes the tube can damage your future ability to conceive.

Women on the Pill also significantly cut their chances of getting known fertility destroyers, including PID, ovarian and endometrial cancer, ovarian cysts, and endometriosis. Plus, they're less likely to develop anemia, rheumatoid arthritis, or breast cysts.

Fertility risks: Once you go off the Pill, chances are you'll resume your pre-Pill menstrual rhythms with few variations. If you had regular periods before, they'll probably be regular again. If not, you can expect the same irregularities, along with any fertility problems you already had.

More disconcerting is the amount of time it sometimes takes for periods to reappear. Because the Pill scrambles brain–ovary communication channels, unscrambling them doesn't always happen quickly. Most women need 2 to 3 months to return to a normal cycle, although fertility can pick up right where it left off—and with heightened vigor. In fact, conception ability may actually peak for some women during the first ovulation after stopping the Pill, and success rates for in vitro fertilization may also rise in the first two post-Pill menstrual cycles.

On the flip side, though, your period may not come back for 6 months or more, although this is a rare occurrence affecting only 1 to 2 percent of women and it has not been determined that the delay is caused by the Pill. (Recall that women whose cycles were irregular before Pill use will most likely have irregular cycles after they stop taking the Pill.)

Giving your ovaries a periodic break from the Pill by using it intermittently may sound like a way to minimize this fertility lag, but there's little evidence that it works. "Don't take a rest from the Pill unless you want to get pregnant," advises Amy Gilbert, M.D., medical director of the Family Tree Clinic in St. Paul, Minnesota, who also teaches in the family and community medicine program at Regent's Hospital there.

After you go off the Pill, deciding how long to wait before trying to conceive is a personal choice. Because of age, you may want to get going immediately. Or you may opt for time to prepare physically and emotionally for pregnancy and parenthood. (You can read about one woman who waited 12 months to conceive after going off birth control so that she could rev up her body and mind for the changes ahead in "A Year's Hiatus after Going Off the Pill Got Her in Top Shape—Physically and Mentally.")

"We usually tell a woman to wait 2 or 3 months before trying to get

WHAT WORKED FOR US

A YEAR'S HIATUS AFTER GOING OFF THE PILL GOT HER IN TOP SHAPE—PHYSICALLY AND MENTALLY

When Marla Hardee Milling and her husband decided to try for a baby, her doctor recommended that she wait 3 months after going off the Pill to allow her menstrual cycles a few complete run-throughs first. But Marla, who'd suffered from Hodgkin's disease a decade earlier, felt particularly uneasy about possible birth defects and pregnancy complications from the Pill's lingering hormonal effects. And though she was 33 with an established public relations career, she still didn't feel fully prepared for the emotional and physical demands of pregnancy and motherhood. Even after her pharmacist suggested waiting at least 6 months, she still wasn't convinced it was long enough.

That's when she hit on the idea of a year-long hiatus to fully prep her body—and mind—for the physical, psychological, and spiritual changes ahead. "For me, that year was about more than just being off the Pill," she recalls. "I used the time to prepare for pregnancy. I tried to imagine what it would be like to have a child and whether I had enough patience. I also tried to get a lot of things out of my system so I wouldn't look back after the baby and regret not having done them."

For the next 12 months, she and her husband indulged in "selfish" pleasures. They stayed up late and skipped work now and then for fun, and enjoyed dining in elegant, intimate restaurants.

"I went off the Pill in January and when the next January came around, I felt ready and relaxed and got pregnant right away," Marla recalls. "Taking time for myself might have even contributed to my getting pregnant so fast."

pregnant—not to get the chemicals out of her bloodstream (they're out in a few days)—but because we like to see what her cycles look like off the Pill so we know when she ovulates and can date the pregnancy," explains Ross Black, M.D., associate clinical professor in the department of family medicine at Northeastern Ohio Universities College of Medicine in Rootstown and a family physician in Cuyahoga Falls, Ohio. "It also gives women time to start taking folic acid before conception and get prepared."

A more serious threat to your fertility is the fact that oral contraceptives may elevate your risk of cervical cancer if you take them for more than 5 years. In addition, fertility threats like diabetes, obesity, and uterine fibroids are sometimes aggravated by the Pill. If you're not happy with the type of pill you're taking, talk to your doctor about low-dose pills, which may have fewer side effects, or progestin-only pills.

Pill use can also cause fertility-robbing nutritional deficiencies. In addition to eating a balanced diet, take a multivitamin for added nutritional insurance. The one you choose should contain a full complement of B vitamins, especially folic acid, which is significantly depleted by the Pill. (See chapter 3 for more fertility-boosting nutrition tips.)

INJECTABLES

Depo-Provera. This birth control method requires a visit to your doctor every 3 months for an injection into your arm or buttock. Like the minipill, it contains progestin, which helps to stop monthly ovulation, thickens cervical mucus, and prevents implantation of fertilized eggs in the uterus.

Fertility benefits: Depo-Provera offers similar fertility protections as the minipill, with one added bonus: Because you're likely to lose your period altogether (a welcome break for some and a not-so-welcome loss of female identity for others), your risk for fertility-threatening disorders caused by regular bleeding, such as iron-deficiency anemia, also decrease.

Fertility risks: Besides not defending against STDs, Depo-Provera may also prompt a Pill-like delay in ovulation that can last anywhere from 3 months to a year or more after the last injection. "This is a long-acting drug," notes Dr. Gilbert. "The longer you use it, the longer it takes to ovulate."

"If you want to conceive soon, Depo-Provera is not a good birth control method for you," adds Andrew M. Kaunitz, M.D., assistant chair of the obstetrics and gynecology department at the University of Florida Health Science Center in Jacksonville.

Lunelle. Launched in 2001, this new arrival contains estrogen and progestin and is given as a monthly shot in your arm, buttock, or thigh by your doctor to stop ovulation, similar to the combined Pill.

Fertility benefits: Similar to the combined Pill.

Fertility risks: Similar to the combined Pill. Regular ovulation usually resumes after 1 to 3 months, but it can take as long as a year.

IMPLANTS

Norplant. This method works by slowly releasing progestin into your body via six matchstick-sized rods that are inserted in your upper arm, under the skin. Like the minipill, it thickens cervical mucus, slowing down sperm and interfering with implantation of a fertilized egg, but it's active for up to 5 years.

Note: Norplant is no longer being marketed because some doctors had trouble removing implants, but many women will continue wearing active Norplant rods until they expire in the months and years to come. Watch for a new single-rod 3-year implant called Implanon, which has fertility benefits and risks similar to Norplant.

Fertility benefits: Similar to the minipill.

Fertility risks: As with the minipill, you may notice a delay in ovulation after the implants are removed.

"Norplant's manufacturer says the hormone is out of your system in 3 days," Dr. Black notes. "But you're not necessarily going to get pregnant right away, because you don't ovulate while you're using it." Menstrual cycles can take 3 months or more to begin again, he adds.

IUDS

Copper IUD. This is a small T-shaped piece of plastic that a doctor inserts into the uterus. While no one fully understands how it works, the arms of the device contain a small amount of copper, which is slowly released into the uterus, preventing egg implantation there. Like other IUDs, it does not protect against ectopic pregnancy, which occurs in the fallopian tubes. It's effective for up to 10 years.

In the 1970s, the Dalkon Shield IUD was linked to PID and infertility caused by blocked fallopian tubes. Millions of women swore off IUDs forever. But new research suggests that the modern copper IUD doesn't boost your risk of infertility or PID (except in the first month after insertion), particularly if you are monogamous and not at risk for STDs.

Fertility benefits: If you don't want the longer fertility disruptions of hormonal birth control methods, IUDs offer a potent alternative. "IUDs have gotten a bad rap," Dr. Gilbert notes. "I'm a big fan of them, and they're immediately reversible. When you want to get pregnant, you just have your doctor pull on the string and remove it."

Note: Many doctors advise waiting a month before trying to conceive because the uterus may continue responding as though the IUD is still there, possibly boosting your chances of a miscarriage if you get pregnant.

Finally, IUDs offer another important fertility benefit as well—a lowered risk of endometrial and cervical cancer.

Fertility risks: The IUD's biggest drawback is that it doesn't protect against fertility-destroying STDs. Also, in rare cases, an IUD can puncture the uterine wall during insertion or cause an infection. And when pregnancies occur—a rarity because IUDs are almost 100 percent effective—they're more likely to be ectopic.

Hormone-releasing IUDs. Approved for use in the United States in 2000, the Mirena intrauterine system is only the latest example of a cross between a copper IUD and hormonal contraceptives. Inserted like a copper IUD, Mirena acts similarly to keep sperm out of the womb, but it also acts hormonally on the reproductive system, like the minipill, via a daily low dose of levonorgestrel. Plus, it's effective for 5 years.

Fertility benefits: Mirena provides all the fertility bonuses of other IUDs, and it decreases your chances of iron deficiency by curtailing bloodflow during your periods, sometimes stopping them altogether.

Fertility risks: Like other IUDs, Mirena doesn't defend against STDs. In addition, like oral contraceptives, it blocks brain–ovary messages, so it may take up to a year for you to conceive after removal. "This isn't the most practical contraceptive choice if you want to get pregnant soon," Dr. Kaunitz says.

VAGINAL RING

NuvaRing. This is a low-dose estrogen- and progestin-releasing ring that you insert into your vagina for 3 weeks and remove during the fourth. It works like a low-dose combined Pill.

Fertility benefits: Similar to the combined Pill.

Fertility risks: Similar to the combined Pill.

FROM CONTRACEPTION . . . TO CONCEPTION

Modern technology offers us numerous birth control choices that are highly effective at preventing pregnancy and, in the case of male and female condoms, sexually transmitted diseases. But if you want to become pregnant at some point in the near future, it's wise to also consider the amount of time it typically takes to return to normal fertility after using each method. Here's a comparison chart to help you make an informed decision about the contraception choice that's best for you. (Keep in mind, though, that the figures below are averages; some women's bodies may take longer to respond.)

Contraceptive	Average Time until Fertility Returns after Stopping Use
Oral contraceptives	1 to 3 months
Depo-Provera	3 to 18 months
Lunelle	1 to 3 months
Implants	1 to 3 months
Copper intrauterine device (IUD)	Within 1 month
Hormone-releasing IUDs	1 to 3 months
Vaginal ring	1 to 3 months
Contraceptive patch	1 to 3 months
Barrier methods	Immediate
Fertility awareness methods	Immediate

CONTRACEPTIVE PATCH

Ortho Evra. Ortho Evra is a self-administered patch that's usually worn on the hip and changed weekly for 3 weeks, then not worn on the fourth. It releases a daily dose of estrogen and progestin, similar to the low-dose combined Pill.

Fertility benefits: Similar to the combined Pill.

Fertility risks: Similar to the combined Pill.

ABOUT FACE

What if you finally meet Mr. Wonderful but he's had a vasectomy? Or you decide you want a baby with husband number two after your tubes are tied? Is there any way to "undo" the undoable?

Well, that depends on how long ago you had the procedure and how it was done, says Ross Black, M.D., associate clinical professor in the department of family medicine at Northeastern Ohio Universities College of Medicine in Rootstown and a family physician in Cuyahoga Falls, Ohio. Fortunately, many "irreversible" tubal ligations and vasectomies are not only reversible, but the surgery to undo them may leave you with reproductive odds that are equal to or better than those you'd get with assisted reproduction techniques. "The success rate for both types of reversals is about 60 to 80 percent," Dr. Black notes.

To undo a vasectomy, your doctor will microsurgically reconnect the two ends of the vas deferens, which were clipped during the original procedure. Called a vasovasostomy, this procedure allows sperm to travel once again from the testes to the penis for ejaculation.

If there's scarring or swelling in the passageway linking the vas deferens and the epididymis (a tube-like coil that collects sperm from the testes and shepherds it out to the vas deferens), your doctor may instead perform a vasoepididy-mostomy. This involves stitching one end of the vas deferens directly to the epididymis and bypassing the troublesome entryway.

Vasectomy reversals cost anywhere from $1,600 to $5,000. Success rates vary and depend on factors like whether your body has developed sperm-destroying antibodies. About one-half to three-quarters of men who undergo vasovasostomy eventually achieve pregnancy with their partners. Men who

---

BARRIER METHODS

Condoms (both male and female), diaphragms, sponges, the cervical cap, and spermicides. All of these devices work by blocking sperm before they reach the womb.

Fertility benefits: Barrier methods aren't the potent pregnancy roadblocks that other birth control options are (you must remember to use them—and use them correctly—every time you have sex), but their fertility

---

receive a vasoepididymostomy achieve pregnancy only about 20 percent of the time.

Your odds for a successful reversal procedure decrease as more time elapses from the date of the original vasectomy. You have a three-in-four chance of pregnancy when less than 3 years has passed. Your odds drop to 50 percent after 3 to 8 years and down to 30 percent after 15 or more years. Keep in mind, too, that it can typically take between 1 and 2 years for pregnancy to occur after a reversal. If vasectomy reversal fails, another option is to collect sperm directly from the epididymis for use during in vitro fertilization.

Reversing a tubal ligation is a more complicated procedure, typically requiring major abdominal surgery to microsurgically sew the fallopian tubes back together so eggs can travel from the ovaries to the womb for fertilization. (There are, however, currently a few surgeons who can do the procedure using a laparoscope, making it outpatient surgery.) In contrast, reversing a vasectomy requires only a small incision in the scrotum.

"A tubal reversal is less difficult than reversing a vasectomy because the tubes are bigger," Dr. Black notes. "But you typically have to stay in the hospital because it's intra-abdominal surgery, and it's very costly." Fees run about $10,000 for the surgeon and considerably more for the hospital stay. Neither is covered by insurance.

Your odds of getting pregnant after a reversal depend on how much of your fallopian tubes were damaged and the training and skill of the surgeon. Whether your tubes were blocked with a clip or ring or cauterized (burned), you have a 75 to 88 percent chance of getting pregnant if you have more than 5 centimeters of tube remaining.

advantages are considerable. Because they don't involve hormonal disruptions to your reproductive system or long-term insertion in the uterus, conception can happen as soon as you put them away.

Male condoms have the added benefit of helping to protect against STDs, including HIV. In fact, short of abstinence, they're the only really reliable way to thwart most infections. Female condoms provide some defense, but not as much.

Fertility risks: Accidental pregnancy is more likely; if bad timing would be disastrous, you might want to consider more reliable options.

NATURAL CONTRACEPTION AND FERTILITY AWARENESS METHODS

Natural contraception methods work on the idea that women are fertile only a few days each month and don't need round-the-cycle contraception. By avoiding sex on or around the time of ovulation or using another contraceptive method on fertile days, such as condoms or a diaphragm, you can prevent pregnancy.

Mucus-monitoring methods are among the most common forms of natural contraception. These require a woman to note changes in the quantity and quality of her cervical mucus, which can give her important clues about when she's likely to be ovulating.

Another common form is the basal body temperature (BBT) method, where a woman records her daily temperature fluctuations. Body temperature will drop slightly, then rise with the production of progesterone. Monthly charting of these changes helps determine when ovulation occurs; after several months, you should have a pretty good idea of when you're fertile, so you'll know what days to avoid having sex or to use other contraceptive methods. Sometimes BBT and mucus-monitoring methods are used in conjunction with one another and called the symptothermal method.

"I think natural contraception is a wonderful method," Dr. Gilbert notes. "It involves both partners and teaches you a lot about your body and tuning in to your cycles."

Fertility benefits: Because you're not using hormones or a physical barrier to block ovulation or egg fertilization, natural contraception methods have the lowest fertility impact on your system. Stop practicing, and you're ready to conceive. Indeed, knowing when you're likely to be ovulating can actually boost your conception odds considerably. (Chapter 12 discusses using fertility awareness methods to improve your chances of getting pregnant.)

Fertility risks: Not only won't you get STD protection, but if you aren't properly trained and don't calculate ovulation exactly, you may find yourself unexpectedly pregnant.

9

Protecting Your Environment
to Protect Your Fertility

It's every mother's wholehearted hope to bring her baby into the most perfect world possible. From the most billowy blankets to the most gentle soap, we earnestly try to create conditions as pure and safe as our wombs. Yet even mothers with the best of intentions feed their newborns poisons.

An American woman's breast milk is likely to be laced with more than 50 industrial chemicals, including a sinister cocktail of pesticides, arsenic, dry-cleaning chemicals, paint fumes, formaldehyde, gasoline additives, and dioxins. And because it's stored in our fatty tissues—where pesticides tend to accumulate—breast milk is even infused with a number of toxicants so hazardous they were banned 20 years ago.

The point isn't to give up breastfeeding—after all, formula contains other contaminants and lacks mom's natural antibodies. But this is one startling example of why it's critical to consider the well-being of your environment, not only during your pregnancy but also during the years leading up to it. Unfortunately, this doesn't simply mean that you should reconsider your job if you work at a toxic chemical factory or put out the "for sale" sign if you live next to an industrial park. Fertility-robbing chemicals can be found in virtually every home, workplace, and community.

Chemicals known as *ovotoxicants*, meaning that they can disrupt a woman's menstrual cycle and even stop ovulation, are found everywhere from beauty salons to rayon factories. More acute exposures to certain ovotoxicants can actually destroy a woman's lifetime supply of eggs. VCH chemicals (used in the manufacture of rubber tires, plastics, and pesticides) as well as PAHs (the hydrocarbons released from cigarettes, auto emissions, and road and roof tar) are being studied for possibly causing premature menopause.

Then there are the heavy metals, industrial chemicals, and other poisons that cause birth defects or developmental delays in a fetus. Toxicologists classify these materials as *teratogens*, which literally means "monster forming." Many of these same chemicals, and others, are responsible for miscarriage.

Fertility-robbing uterine and ovarian cancer can be traced to environmental hazards categorized as *carcinogens*. Suspicious substances are found everywhere from contaminated drinking water to decomposing vinyl floors to personal care products. Other fertility-compromising conditions, such as endometriosis and polycystic ovary syndrome or PCOS (otherwise known as Stein–Leventhal disease), may be aggravated or caused by a growing number of toxicants, called *endocrine-disrupting chemicals* (EDCs), that have been shown to interfere with proper hormone functioning. EDCs are even suspected of nudging girls into earlier and earlier puberty, which in itself can be linked to early menopause, cancer, or conditions such as endometriosis and PCOS.

ENVIRONMENTAL HEALTH IS A GUY'S RESPONSIBILITY, TOO

In the 1970s, a group of wives talking at a baseball game found out they had a lot in common. As their husbands were concentrating on striking out their coworkers, the women realized they were all striking out when it came to getting pregnant.

The men all worked in a chemical plant that manufactured the compound dibromochloropropane (DBCP), which was used as a fumigant against fruit pests. These couples' fertility problems were explained when a formal study revealed that out of 24 men in their division at the plant, half had low sperm count or couldn't produce sperm at all. A follow-up study on 142 DBCP workers confirmed that the longer a man is exposed to the compound, the lower the quality of his sperm. As a result of the testing, the Occupational Safety and Health Administration (OSHA) and the Environmental Protection Agency (EPA) categorized DBCP as a reproductive toxicant, and it was banned for use on U.S. crops by 1985.

The good news is that some of the men were able to father children after they reduced their exposure to DBCP. Still, other men suffered permanent damage to the cells in their testes that produce sperm, rendering them sterile.

"The DBCP workers' experience really brought forth the understanding that a man can also be exposed to toxicants that can affect his ability to have children," notes reproductive toxicologist Steve Schrader, Ph.D. As the chief of the reproductive health assessment section at the National Institute for Occupational Safety and Health, Dr. Schrader spends most of his time studying hazards to male fertility in the workplace. Besides DBCP, he's found that numerous other pesticides, solvent chemicals like glycol ethers, and lead fit the criteria of *spermatotoxicants*, agents that decrease sperm count or quality, and *testicular toxicants*, substances that actually damage the cells in the organs where sperm are produced.

"On the brighter side, as long as men are still producing *some* sperm, provided those sperm are healthy, men can still bring about conception. But a guy has more reason for concern if his wife is near the end of her childbearing years, because lower sperm count clearly figures into the time it takes to conceive," explains reproductive epidemiologist Shanna H. Swan, Ph.D., research professor in the department of family and community medicine at the University of Missouri–Columbia.

Experts like Dr. Swan suspect that the same environmental factors that could be compromising sperm quality could be contributing to the 1.5 to

3 percent annual increase in testicular and prostate cancer among American and European men since the 1970s.

In addition, men exposed to hormone-disrupting chemicals may be experiencing problems similar to those of the Lake Apopka alligators. After pesticides were accidentally spilled in the Florida lake in 1980, testosterone in male alligators plummeted to the levels of the female gators. Even 20 years after the accident, many of their penises are too shrunken for procreation.

Similarly, human male fetuses exposed to hormone-disrupting chemicals are more likely to develop genital deformities. In fact, Dr. Swan and her colleagues theorize that abnormalities in genital development, declining sperm count, and testicular cancer may be part of one syndrome all related to exposure to hormone-disrupting chemicals.

KNOW YOUR RISKS

Trying to avoid all the toxicants in our environment is like trying to avoid a mosquito bite while hiking through a steamy swamp in a bikini. Our workplaces, homes, and communities are swarming with any of the 152,000 potentially toxic substances listed in the federal Registry of Toxic Effects of Chemical Substances. Fortunately, with the exception of a highly toxic chemical spill or workplace accident, one bite (or toxic exposure) isn't usually the problem. Doctors are more concerned with a person's overall "body burden." "When it comes to low-grade chemicals like those in household products, it's not that one exposure can threaten someone's fertility, but the fact that a person is exposed to so many different chemicals so much of the time," explains reproductive endocrinologist and gynecologic surgeon Deborah Metzger, M.D., Ph.D., medical director of Helena Women's Health in San Jose, California, and medical advisor to this book.

"Reducing toxic exposures requires awareness and lifestyle modifications. Don't assume that governmental regulatory agencies are sufficiently protecting you," cautions Ted Schettler, M.D., M.P.H., science director of

The Science and Environmental Health Network and an internist at Boston Medical Center. He is the coauthor of two books on the topic, *Generations at Risk* and *In Harm's Way*.

Chemicals are not regulated in the same strict manner that medications are. The FDA tests each medication and won't release it to the public until all the safety studies have been reviewed, but this doesn't happen with chemicals. Furthermore, "information about reproductive hazards has rarely been used in setting workplace exposure levels," note public statements by OSHA, the government body that enforces workplace standards. Similarly, the FDA requires that the personal care products Americans use in their everyday routines be tested and labeled only for little more than skin irritation.

Essentially, a chemical can be manufactured liberally until what's called "proof of harm" is demonstrated. Unfortunately, history is replete with reasons to take better precaution up front, says Dr. Swan. For instance, it took 50 years to ban organochlorine pollutants like the chemical-warfare-agent-turned-pesticide DDT and polychlorinated biphenyl chemicals (PCBs), which were widely used in electric transformers. By the time these organochlorines were recognized as potential human carcinogens, with toxic effects on the endocrine and reproductive systems, they had made their way into the soil, surface water, air, plants, and animal tissue *in all regions of the earth*.

Today, we're still discovering negative effects of PCBs and DDT. Not only do they continue to show up in human breast milk, but the developing fetus may still receive enough lingering residues to lower its future IQ.

For both personal lifestyle decisions and regulatory decisions by the government, visionaries in the field of medicine, science, and government suggest applying the "precautionary principle"—a concept that grew out of Germany's Green Movement. "When there's possible long-term harm to humans or the environment, the idea is to act to prevent damage rather than to try to clean up after the fact, when it may be too late," explains Dr. Schettler.

So that you can take appropriate precautions, we'll outline some major groups of potential hazards. Following that, we'll offer some specific actions for lowering your exposure to these hazards in your workplace, home, and community.

Organic Solvents and VOCs

Organic solvents are petroleum-based liquids that are prized for their industrial use of dissolving other substances. They're used in industries as diverse as auto repair, electronics, dry cleaning, health care, photography, printing, agriculture, furniture building, construction, and cosmetology, to name a few. Household products contain them as well, including glues, markers, correction fluids, paints, personal care products, and some cleaning agents. Consequently, humans are exposed to complex mixtures of solvents on a daily basis. Since organic solvents evaporate at room temperature, they have a particularly easy time entering the human body: We simply inhale them as we breathe. In this form, they are known as *volatile organic compounds* (VOCs).

Several studies from Finland and the United States observed that women who had miscarriages were two to four times more likely to be exposed to organic solvents at work compared to women who carried to term. Another study showed a 75 percent decrease in fertility among women occupationally exposed to organic solvents. And 20 years' worth of data on men who attended a Canadian fertility clinic indicate a proportional relationship between solvent exposure intensity and sperm count decline.

Of course, all solvents are not equally hazardous, Dr. Schrader points out. The solvent chemicals most well-established as a reproductive hazard are the glycol ethers, which cause testicular atrophy at high exposures. They are prevalent in brake fluid, ink, paint, varnish, photography chemicals, circuit board production, perfumes, and cosmetics. Other solvents thoroughly documented as reproductive hazards are perchloroethylene (a dry-cleaning chemical), toluene (used in glues, inks, paints, and gasoline), and trihalomethanes (a by-product of chlorinated tap water). Because of its high accumulation in the average home, the solvent formaldehyde is also a cause for concern. It has been well-documented as a cause of menstrual irregularity and is also linked to miscarriage.

Agricultural Agents

Pesticides are a key area in which doctors and environmentalists wish that the precautionary principle were applied more often. It took tragic effects on human health and wildlife to ban poisons such as DDT, chlordane, arsenic, dieldrin, aldrin, and endrin. Still, more than 600 pesticides are registered for use today. Of the chemicals manufactured in particularly high volume (in excess of one million pounds a year), 19 are listed on the EPA's Toxics Release Inventory because of reproductive or developmental toxicity. The many classes of pesticides and their qualities are too extensive to list here, but pesticides in general should be suspected as potential carcinogens, teratogens, spermatotoxicants, endocrine disruptors, and general health hazards.

Austrian researchers found that men experiencing infertility were 10 times more often employed in jobs related to agriculture or pesticides than fertile men. Numerous studies also note an increased rate of spontaneous abortions and stillbirths in female agricultural workers. Of course, it's not only farm workers who are exposed to pesticides on a daily basis. Americans go through 70 million pounds of insecticides, herbicides, and fungicides a year for home, lawn, and garden use. Pesticides are also applied liberally to public spaces like golf courses.

When it comes to animal farming, beef cows are routinely dosed with anabolic steroid hormones to force them to "bulk up" quicker. The hormone of choice in the livestock industry was at one time DES—the same synthetic estrogen agent that mothers took to supposedly prevent miscarriage in the 1950s and 1960s. DES was banned after it proved to have the opposite effect—not only did it *cause* miscarriage, but children who survived developed malformed reproductive systems and, in some cases, vaginal cancer.

Not only are hormones similar to DES still used in beef production today, but in 1993, the Monsanto chemical company began to mass-market the recombinant bovine growth hormone (rbGH) to increase dairy cows' milk supply. Approximately 30 percent of American dairy cows receive the protein-forming hormones.

"There's no question that residues of these hormones make their way into commercial milk and meat, but the FDA only permits the sale of food with residue levels they consider safe," says Dr. Schettler. Applying their precautionary principle, Europeans refuse hormone-raised animal products, claiming uncertain health outcomes and environmental concerns (such as hormones from the animals' urine leeching into the water supply).

Dioxins

Dioxins are truly renegade chemicals. No industry intentionally produces them, but they are a by-product of pesticide production, plastic manufacturing, and the pulp and paper industry. Like DDT and PCBs, dioxins have the sinister talent for bioaccumulating in the ecosystem. The World Health Organization recognizes them as carcinogens, and they are considered endocrine-disrupting chemicals by the Environmental Protection Agency.

When some members of a colony of female rhesus monkeys (whose reproductive system is remarkably similar to that of human women) were given low doses of the dioxin TCDD, 79 percent of the exposed monkeys eventually developed endometriosis. The monkeys who weren't given the dioxin were much less likely to develop endometriosis. Researchers noted that the severity of endometriosis was directly proportional to the amount of dioxin the monkey was given—yet even the most severe cases were exposed to half of the levels encountered by the general human population. Leading to increased destruction of sperm and eggs as well as blockages and scar tissue in the female reproductive tract, endometriosis is largely responsible for the 600,000 hysterectomies performed a year. (See chapters 15 and 17 for more information on the endometriosis–infertility link.)

Because of the remote chance of dioxin residues, the Endometriosis Association urges consumers to avoid chlorine-bleached feminine hygiene products—and to boycott chlorine-bleached paper products. (If pads and tampons don't specifically say that they aren't bleached with chlorine, you can assume that they are.) Suppliers of nonchlorinated hygiene products are listed in the Environmentally Friendly Companies section on page 323.

Plastics and Their Additives

Plastics are fundamentally problematic because of the pollutants—including dioxins and other harsh organochlorines—generated during their production, as well as their mammoth contribution to the waste stream, says Dr. Schettler. Another worry is that additives that give plastics their different qualities, like flexibility, may leech into common products, such as food, bottled water, and personal care products, causing ill effects. For example, the additive bisphenol A has a number of adverse effects on the reproductive system of research animals, including decreased sperm production in males and abnormally elevated estrogen levels in females. While the FDA allows 50 parts per billion (ppb) to leech into food, even levels between 2 and 20 ppb caused a 20 percent sperm reduction in animal studies. Two billion pounds of bisphenol A are produced each year to make food containers and baby bottles and to line metal cans.

Phthalates, the most common of the plasticizers, are also used for food containers and some brands of cling wrap. Their main use, though, is to make the PVC plastic popular for vinyl flooring, packaging, and medical supplies such as IV bags. At high levels, phthalates are associated with miscarriage and testicular toxicity. Even at relatively lower levels, phthalates appear to alter estrogen and androgen levels. A recent report from the Centers for Disease Control and Prevention stated that levels of phthalates in people in the United States, particularly women of reproductive age, were higher than expected. The levels the scientists found were within the same range that causes reproductive defects in mice.

Other potentially hazardous plasticizers include *adipates*, which can be teratogens, as well as *nonyl phenol* and *organotins*, which both appear to be endocrine disruptors. In terms of leeching, all plastics are not created equal, comments Dr. Schettler. It's easier for additives to leech out of PVC plastic because they aren't bonded to the polymer in PVC. Additives are less likely to leech from polyethylene (marked with the recycling symbol #4) and polyurethane.

Heavy Metals

It's not so difficult to understand how synthetic, industrial chemicals could be threatening our health. But could elements that occur naturally in the earth's crust also be health hazards? According to experts, the answer is yes. The concern, though, lies in the *excess* of metals like lead and mercury that have become ubiquitous in the environment through worldwide mining, processing, and their use in everyday products.

Lead was essentially the first known reproductive toxicant. As early as 1860, scientists noticed that the wives of lead workers were less likely to become pregnant, and those who did were more likely to have miscarriages. Lead has clearly antagonistic effects on male reproduction as a testicular toxicant and a spermatotoxicant (in fact, it was once an active ingredient in commercial spermicides). Furthermore, the neurological and behavioral development of a child who was exposed to lead as a fetus may be permanently impaired. Since its ill effects to the health of a developing fetus or child are unquestionable, lead has been banned for use nationwide in gasoline and commercial canning. But dangerous exposure still results from old paint, lead pipes, and the residues from past uses that have accumulated in soil.

When mercury reaches toxic levels, it may disrupt menstrual cycles or cause thyroid damage. Even long-term exposure at levels lower than what is considered toxic is suspected of hormone disruption. "This is one reason why I believe people should ask their dentists for alternatives to silver-mercury fillings, which can leech into the bloodstream," says Howard Buttram, M.D., a board-certified expert in environmental and internal medicine who practices the Foresight Program for Preconception Care at The Woodlands Healing Research Center in Quakertown, Pennsylvania. If a new cavity is discovered, you may be able to have it filled with porcelain. Unfortunately, the process of removing an old metal filling can *really* release the mercury, so most doctors will tell you to leave a metal mouth as it is.

Like lead, mercury's damage to a developing fetus's brain is well-established. Mercury is well-distributed throughout air, water, and soil, and it can accumulate to toxic levels in fish. It continues to be used industrially for fluorescent lighting, electrical equipment, and agriculture.

Manganese makes its way into the atmosphere through the manufacture of dry-cell batteries, iron and steel products, and certain paints and agrochemicals. It's also found in gasoline fumes treated with the antiknock agent manganese tricarbonyl. One study documents that workers were significantly less fertile when exposed to just one-fifth of the allowable workplace levels of manganese dust or vapor.

In women, cadmium may trigger decreased production of the hormone needed to maintain a pregnancy, human chorionic gonadotropin. And though the heavy metal arsenic has the legacy of being highly toxic, it was once widely distributed because of its commercial use as a wood preservative and as a pesticide. Both uses are now banned, but it's still present in treated wood, drinking water, and body fat. Hungarian researchers found that people living in an area of arsenic-contaminated water had higher levels of miscarriage and stillbirth.

KEEP YOURSELF SAFE AT WORK

As the former director of safety, health, and environmental affairs at the world's largest ethylene oxide handling facility, Mary DeVany took all the recommended precautions to protect herself from the chemical manufactured to sterilize medical equipment. Despite carefully staying under the 1,000 parts per million (ppm) exposure limit, she endured three miscarriages between her first and second child. Soon after, the government-mandated standard exposure level to ethylene oxide dropped dramatically from 1,000 ppm down to 1 ppm. Ethylene oxide became one of only three toxicants with OSHA exposure limits created specifically for reproductive hazards.

"We now know ethylene oxide can cause increased miscarriage rates for women, as well as two-headed sperm, sperm that can't swim, and, eventually, male sterility," remarks DeVany, who currently works as an industrial hygiene consultant helping organizations comply with OSHA and EPA regulations.

The lesson: Even when exposure standards are maintained, safety isn't guaranteed. "My general recommendation is to expose yourself to chemicals as little as possible whether there is an accepted exposure limit or not," DeVany says. And whatever your profession, follow universal safety practices such as frequent handwashing and proper ventilation—even if the material you work with seems relatively innocuous, she advises.

Here are some additional guidelines for staying safe on the job.

Act like any material you work with is toxic, whether it is known to be or not. Food service workers, custodians, cosmetologists, dry cleaners, and artists may all be exposed to reproductive hazards as potent as those affecting people who work in more industrial professions and laboratories. Even office workers should keep their workspace as far as possible from copy machines, fax machines, and other chemical sources.

Check the material safety data sheet on the material you work with. Under federal law, chemical manufacturers are required to develop these information reports on hazardous materials they produce or import, and employers are required to make them available to workers. If reproductive hazards have been reported on a material, it will be listed under "health effects."

If you need more information on a substance, consult a teratogen information service. The Organization of Teratology Information Services (OTIS) is a nonprofit group with the sole purpose of providing information on the effect that drugs, medications, and chemicals may have on a fetus or potential fetus. An OTIS spokesperson will answer your question over the phone from one of the satellite offices, which are located all over the United States and Canada. Call the main OTIS line at (866) 626-6847 or log on to www.otispregnancy.org.

Seek out an expert. If you want still more information on a reproductive hazard, or think you may be exposed to a harmful substance, consult a health care professional in the occupational health field, recommends

DeVany. An occupational health nurse, occupational physician, or toxicologist will know what to test for and can also advise you on filing claims specifically related to reproductive hazards. The next best authority would be your company's safety, health, and environmental manager employed by the human resources department, DeVany says. To find an expert, contact the American Academy of Environmental Medicine (see page 316 for their contact information).

Take these three standard steps. If it turns out that you are working with a hazardous substance, the first thing you want to do is substitute a less toxic material whenever possible. Occupational health experts can help you identify alternative materials. Second, if there is no substitute, it's essential that the highest standards are being met for containment, ventilation, and personal protective equipment, says DeVany. Third, put limits on the time you are exposed. "When workers must be knowingly exposed to finite amounts of hazardous material, it's generally recommended that four people rotate throughout an 8-hour shift, so that no one worker has more than 2 hours of exposure," DeVany says.

Become an expert on your personal protective equipment. Your protective clothing, respirators, gloves, and other safety equipment are your last line of defense against exposure. Experts stress that it's not enough to just use your protective equipment—you need thorough training and understanding of it.

"I conducted a study in the semiconductor industry where women wore full-body coverings and gloves. But it turned out the *chips* were being protected, not the women. The women were inhaling enough of the solvents to cause delayed pregnancy and miscarriage," Dr. Swan recalls. Attend all training sessions, find out what exactly is being protected, and determine whether the correct safety equipment is being matched with the specific chemical you use.

Don't take toxicants home with you. Whenever possible, leave workplace clothing and shoes at your work site, and keep clothing to change into in a place where it won't be exposed, advises Dr. Schrader. If you must bring workplace clothing home to launder, store and wash it separately from your other clothes. If you have to take your shoes home, leave them outside.

Never eat, drink, or smoke where chemicals are used or stored. Food, drinks, and cigarettes might absorb dust or fumes or cause you to ingest hazardous material on your hands. Furthermore, the carbon in cigarettes has an infamous ability to absorb volatile material. Finally, no matter what material you work with, remember to always wash up before eating, smoking, or going home and before and after going to the bathroom.

Know your rights. If an employer is less than willing to correct a potentially dangerous working condition, contact OSHA. This federal agency regulates employee exposure to physical, biological, and chemical hazards. (See page 319 for contact information.)

CREATE A HEALTHIER HOME

When we think of pollution, the image of smokestacks and congested cities comes to mind—not the safe havens we call home. In reality, the air inside most living quarters can be more seriously polluted than the outdoor air in the largest and most industrialized cities and can pose a greater risk to our health, according to the EPA.

"The problem is that our well-insulated homes allow substances to truly linger, combining with other low-grade chemicals in ways that have probably never been studied in a lab," points out Dr. Schettler.

"Two chemicals together may have tenfold greater toxicity than either one individually," adds Dr. Buttram.

To safeguard your health, you need to become an environmentally aware consumer. After all, there's a lot that can be done to lower your toxic load on a day-to-day basis. Here are some examples.

Safely dispose of unnecessary chemicals. Gather up all the partially full containers of old or unneeded chemicals throughout your home. But don't simply toss them in the garbage can, where they can pollute your community, urges the EPA. Most municipalities have hazardous material collections several times a year or can tell you the proper hazardous waste site

(continued on page 140)

DON'T GET GREENWASHED!

Your cabinets are probably stocked with products claiming to be "pure and natural." As if words aren't enough, manufacturers of soaps, lotions, and cleaning products also like to put images of beautiful, windswept fields and pristine waterfalls on their packaging. But since household products aren't required to list all their ingredients (and even if they do, hazardous chemicals may be listed by a commercial name that's difficult to

Suspicious Ingredient	Why It Doesn't Qualify as Pure and Natural	Products to Check
Artificial colors	Serve no other purpose but visual; several formulas like FD&C Red 33 are suspected carcinogens	Soaps, bubble bath, lotions, shampoos
Benzene (includes paradichlorobenzene)	Recognized carcinogen, reproductive toxicant, and teratogen (a substance that causes harm to a developing fetus); suspected endocrine disruptor	Perfumes, degreasers, air fresheners and deodorants,laundry starch, moth repellent, new bathroom rugs
Brominated flame retardants	Potential hormone disruptor	Fabric-based products
Chlorine	Creates by-products of dioxin, a recognized carcinogen, endocrine disruptor, and serious water contaminant	Bleached paper products, coffee filters, feminine hygiene products, cleansers, dishwashing soaps, laundry products
Formaldehyde	Recognized carcinogen; may cause menstrual irregularity	Air fresheners and deodorants, cosmetics, disinfectants, floor polish, rug and upholstery cleaners
Glycol ethers	Recognized reproductive hazards and developmental toxicants	Stain removers, glass cleaners, degreasers, cosmetics, perfumes
N-methyl-2-pyrrolidone (NMP)	Strong potential as a teratogen	Cosmetics

identify), the only way to really know what's in there is to call the manufacturer.

If you use something every day, it's probably worth screening. If you encounter the following ingredients, you may want to reduce your use of the product, or find an alternative that can guarantee that it is *truly* "pure and natural." (A list of companies that offer environmentally friendly products can be found in the Resources section on page 323.)

Suspicious Ingredient	Why It Doesn't Qualify as Pure and Natural	Products to Check
Parabens (may have the prefix *methyl*, *ethyl*, *propyl*, or *butyl*)	Potential hormone disruptors	Cosmetics, antibacterial toothpastes
Phenol (may have the prefix *alkyl* or *bis* and the suffix *ethoxylates*)	Potential hormone disruptor (Alkylphenol ethoxylates have been banned for European personal care products because of a suspicious impact on reproductive health.)	Detergents, disinfectants, mouthwash, medicated skin products
Phosphates	Disrupt the ecology of lakes and streams	Dishwasher detergents, laundry products
Phthalates	Potential testicular toxicants, hormone disruptors, and teratogens	Food packaging made out of paperboard and plastic, plastic food storage containers, cling wrap, cans, baby toys
Propane and butane	Compromise air quality	Aerosol spray products
Talc	Linked to ovarian cancer (when used on genitals); may contain mercury contaminants	Powders, antiperspirants
Toluene	Potential hormone disruptor and teratogen	Nail polish, cleaning products, dyes, glues
Trichloroethylene	Recognized carcinogen and potential hormone disruptor, teratogen, and reproductive toxicant	Rug cleaners, laundry products

to take them to. If your community doesn't have a pickup day, the EPA encourages you to lobby for one!

Filter your drinking *and* bathing water. Pesticide contamination, heavy metals, dioxins, and water treatment by-products are just a few of the reasons to filter your water. Understand, however, that even if you have a filter on your drinking faucet, you get the same amount of contaminants from a shower as if you drank 2 gallons of unfiltered water, Dr. Swan explains. The ideal filter would be at the intake of your house, protecting your whole water supply, including the water you use to wash your dishes and clothes. If that's not an option, you can purchase individual filters for both your sink and showerhead through companies that supply natural products (see Environmentally Friendly Companies on page 323 for contact information). "Of course, filters can do more harm than good when gunk builds up on them, so change them according to the manufacturer's recommendations," advises Dr. Swan.

Practice *true* home improvement. Indoor painting and remodeling should ideally take place during warmer seasons when windows and doors can be open. Follow the manufacturer's directions for paint strippers, aerosol sprays, paints, and other solvents. If you think you've run into old lead paint, the EPA strongly advises you to have it removed professionally—and while you're not at home.

Select safe paint. Your best option is to purchase paints and strippers created for their low environmental impact, such as Safecoat products, which are free of heavy-metal drying agents, formaldehyde, acetone, and harsh preservatives. Safecoat is sold by dealers throughout the United States or can be purchased by mail order direct from the manufacturer. (See Environmentally Friendly Companies on page 323 for contact information.) The next best thing is to replace petroleum-based painting products with water-based varieties, which contain fewer VOCs and don't require turpentine.

Reconsider rugs. Synthetic new carpets come with a concoction of vinyl acetate, isooctane, styrene butadiene, formaldehyde, and 4-phenylcyclohexane—chemicals that are as toxic as they sound. (Vinyl flooring also gives off a wide variety of toxic fumes and dust.) On the other hand, old rugs, no matter how well you vacuum, are traps for heavy metals and pesticides tracked in on your shoes, plus the chemicals you've released in your home. Tile and natural wood floors are the least polluting (and most durable) flooring options, says Dr. Buttram.

If you're set on carpeting, true wool carpets and sometimes wool-synthetic blends are usually untreated because the naturally occurring lanolin offers stain protection. If you can't get untreated carpets, have them unrolled and aired out for as long as possible before they are installed.

Purchase solid wood products whenever possible. Furniture made with plywood, glues, and particleboard has three different sources of formaldehyde. Solid wood, on the other hand, is easy on your air, says Dr. Buttram. If you are doing your own building and must use plywood, the plywood made for outdoor use generally contains fewer VOCs than the indoor variety.

Seek secondhand items. Not only are rescued treasures from yard sales easy on the wallet and waste stream, they may be easier on your home's air. Formaldehyde emissions in new fabrics and furniture generally decrease over time. That also goes for car interiors, adds Dr. Buttram.

Hang out your purchases. Most fabrics, plastic, and other synthetic products purchased today have potent out-gasses. Hang out your purchases for a few days, even if a shower curtain looks funny on your clothesline. The chemicals that don't air out may be baked out by the sun, Dr. Buttram explains.

Filter out air pollution. Reducing your use of pesticides and VOC-emitting products is your first goal. In addition, clean heating, ventilation, and air-conditioning vents; overhead fans; and open windows will help flush out the pollutants you can't prevent. As far as air filters, you'll receive the greatest benefits from heavy-duty HEPA (high-efficiency particulate air) models.

Don't be duped by dry cleaning. Dry cleaning may take the spots out of your clothes, but the mark it could leave on your air quality and health is a serious issue for any couple hoping to conceive. In several studies, both men and women who worked in dry-cleaning businesses took significantly longer to conceive than people who didn't. Even more alarming is the high rate of miscarriages reported in pregnant women who work in or simply *live near* dry cleaners. The main chemical used in the industry, per-chloroethylene, is classified as a possible human carcinogen as well as a spermatotoxicant and ovotoxicant. Even if you don't work or live around dry cleaning, experts are concerned that the chemical may be emitted by your dry-cleaned clothes and urge you to use alternatives.

The simplest solution is to stop buying dry-clean–only apparel. Or, find out if you have an environmentally sensitive cleaner in your area, such as the national chain Hangers Cleaners (they use a carbon dioxide process rather than perchloroethylene). For a list of store locations, visit www.hangersdrycleaners.com.

KEEP YOUR FOOD PURE

It's not like you can taste dioxin in your scallops, see phthalates that might leech into your soup, or smell traces of lead in your broccoli. But once you become aware of what covert reproductive hazards might be associated with the food supply, you won't have to take so many risks.

It used to be that all you had to think about when preparing a meal was if it was nutritious and tasted good. But to be truly proactive, you need to modify your food choices to reduce the amount of agrochemicals, heavy metals, plastic by-products, and other reproductive hazards to which you could be exposed.

Grow your own. The ultimate way to avoid potential pesticide residue, questionable preservatives, and packaging chemicals leeching into your food is to feast from your own garden, points out Dr. Buttram. If you're new to gardening, log on to the Web site www.organicgardening.com for tons of practical advice and to request a trial issue of *OG* magazine. In addition, your local extension service (check the "county" listings in your phone book) can answer many of your garden start-up questions over the phone.

Avoid planting a roadside plot. If you plant in close proximity to a heavily traveled road, your garden may pick up soil residues of lead, mercury, and other car emissions, in addition to roadside weed-killers and pesticides that might be sprayed by your county. If you don't have an alternative location, Dan Sullivan, senior editor of *OG* magazine, suggests switching to container gardening—even if you have to put containers inside the house or on your roof!

Seek certified organic products. "Organic" means food grown without man-made pesticides, chemical fertilizers, antibiotics, or added hormones, and food that is not genetically modified. Since the year 2000, the federal government regulates the use of the term *organic* on food. In order to use the label, farms must prove they've been truly organic for 3 or more years and pass ongoing inspections by certifying agencies.

You may also be lucky enough to have an organic farmer co-op in your community (sometimes called a CSA) that offers you several ways to share in the harvest. Co-ops might involve working in the fields for discounted produce or receiving home delivery of the week's picks. If you can't grow or buy organic food locally, a wide variety of fresh and prepared food can be ordered through national distributors (see Environmentally Friendly Companies on page 323 for details).

Eat in season. In the big picture, the farther your food travels, the greater the stress on the entire environment, considering the transportation and packaging it takes to get it to your door. In addition, out-of-season produce is usually imported, which makes it twice as likely to be contaminated with renegade agrochemicals that were banned for use by U.S. farmers, says Dr. Buttram.

Be a micro-manager. Before popping your next meal into the microwave, be aware that heating makes it easier for plasticizers to leech into your food. This is especially true if you aren't using official microwave containers (plastic margarine tubs and yogurt containers are out). If you have to nuke something covered with plastic wrap, at least make sure the wrap doesn't come in contact with the food, Dr. Buttram stresses. It's also important to dispose of plastic food and drink receptacles and plastic eating utensils when they become well-worn, since wear and tear makes the chemicals they contain more likely to leech into your food.

Store food in glass, not plastic. If you can buy food that comes in glass containers rather than plastic or aluminum, that's ideal. If you can't, the best you can do is to transfer it into glass and ceramic storage containers. It's especially important to do this with meat, cheese, and other fatty products that absorb contaminants more easily (shave off the area touching the plastic before transferring). When storing leftovers, opt for glass or ceramic containers as well.

Be cautious about local fish. Accumulations of dioxin, mercury, PCB, the pesticide toxaphene, and other contaminants that might be in your local bodies of water can earn an EPA fish advisory warning to limit or avoid consumption. The EPA strongly advises you to contact your state fish advisory agency to inquire about current restrictions (they change all the time) before making a meal out of a local catch. By the end of 2000, 41 states issued 2,242 fish advisories for mercury alone. Another 37 states issued 679 advisories for PCBs.

Be selective about commercial fish. When it comes to commercial fish, the FDA has issued a blanket recommendation that pregnant women and women who are planning to get pregnant should stop eating shark, swordfish, king mackerel, and tilefish. This seafood generally harbors the most mercury. Because of tuna's relatively high mercury levels, Dr. Buttram also recommends eating it only once a week. That said, the FDA clarifies that seafood is still good for you. In fact, the agency encourages women to eat 12 ounces of cooked fish a week. The safest policy is to select a wide variety of catches and not consume too much of any one kind.

Trim fat. The first place that contaminants like dioxins, pesticides, hormones, and PCBs accumulate in fish and meat is the fatty portion. Making an effort to trim fat (and skin fish) will help reduce your toxic load.

Don't eat from lead-glazed pottery. As tempting as it is to serve from that brightly colored Mexican bowl, it's best not to eat or drink from any pottery if you have suspicions that the paint or material could be lead-based, says Dr. Buttram.

PROTECT YOUR COMMUNITY

When it comes to protecting your environment against fertility-robbing pollutants, you need to think both big *and* small. While it's clear that the home and workplace can harbor potentially hazardous contaminants, two sources suspected of triggering early menopause as well as low sperm count come from *general* pollution—auto exhaust that lingers in city streets, and the secondhand smoke most of us encounter on a daily basis. In other words, our *common* air, water, and soil have a profound impact on long-term fertility—and can compromise the quality of life for a future child.

Often it's the moms acting on instinct to protect their families—and unborn children—who tackle the issues beyond their own backyards. Lois Gibbs made the daunting discovery that her town's children were sick because her neighborhood was built on 20,000 tons of toxic chemicals. As spokesperson for the Love Canal Homeowners Council, she generated enough national attention to secure the relocation of 700 households and initiate the U.S. Superfund program (the program created to investigate and enforce cleanup of the nation's most severely polluted locations).

"It takes both a narrow and broad concern for your own health, your family's health, your own community, and the global community to close the circle on protecting your reproductive health, while creating a safer world for a future child," Dr. Schettler says. "That doesn't mean you have to do it all, all of the time," he adds. The key is to keep your eye on the whole picture. Here are some pointers for protecting your piece of the globe.

Establish allies. You don't have to be an environmental activist to contribute positively to the health and welfare of your community. Any civic organization is a great way to stay on top of issues and get to know other concerned citizens. Consider attending functions of your local parent–teacher organization, neighborhood association, historical society, or something comparable. If you do need to mobilize against, say, a hazardous landfill proposed in your town, or an overuse of pesticides in your favorite park, you'll have allies already in place.

Track the air and water quality in your area. The EPA Web site (www.epa.gov) can connect you with reports for both water and air quality in your zip code. You can also call the Safe Drinking Water Hotline at (800) 426-4791 for a list of state drinking water offices. Another great resource if you want to learn about the science and politics behind regional and national water issues is Clean Water Action. Their national office can be reached at (202) 895-0420, or you can visit www.cleanwateraction.org.

Take public transportation and car pools. Reducing auto emissions is something tangible you can do on a day-to-day basis to curb heavy metals and hormone-disrupting agents that infiltrate your community.

Invest in the future. Putting your savings in "green funds" is a way to reward companies who make it a priority to reduce pollution and waste rather than supporting corporations who don't. The Social Investment Forum is an international trade organization with financial planners who specialize in funds screened for environmental and other social concerns. Contact them at (202) 872-5319, or visit www.socialinvest.org. You can also review the environmental policies of specific businesses and purchase a "green" investment guide through www.coopamerica.org.

Be a Web watchdog. It's almost too good to be true, but the Environmental Defense's Web site can tell you exactly what companies in your zip code release chemical emissions and how much. (You can then look up each chemical to see if it has any reproductive toxicity.) Another page reveals the status of any Superfund site or hazardous waste facility in your community. You can even send letters to government representatives asking for action, directly through the same Web site. This powerful resource is at www.scorecard.org.

10

Avoiding Fertility-Threatening Illness and Medical Treatment

Imagine undergoing an emergency appendectomy one night after waking with severe abdominal pain. Or finding a cancerous lump in your breast that requires several immediate rounds of chemotherapy.

Thanks to modern medicine, your chances of surviving either one are good. What you may not know, though—and what your doctor might not tell you—is that your fertility could be wiped out in the process. Indeed, many surgeries and drug treatments, not to mention infections and chronic diseases such as diabetes and high blood pressure, can do significant reproductive harm to you and your partner—sometimes years before you're ready to start a family. The result: future fertility frustrations and pregnancy complications, if you do manage to conceive.

That's why educating yourself now is so vital. You may not be able to ward off every infection or avoid needed surgical procedures, but in most cases, you and your partner can take steps to lessen their impact on your reproductive future.

When it comes to preserving your fertility, "it's really important to find a doctor who will talk to you," advises G. David Adamson, M.D., a reproductive endocrinologist who is director of Fertility Physicians of

Northern California in San Jose and Palo Alto and clinical professor at Stanford University School of Medicine. Be sure your doctor informs you of all your treatment options, and have him list any potential fertility threats associated with each choice.

CONTROL CHRONIC CONDITIONS

The male and female reproductive systems are engineering marvels. To function optimally, both rely on an exquisite balance of precisely timed hormonal messages and the peak performance of the reproductive organs. Unfortunately, a chronic health condition such as diabetes or thyroid disease can sometimes snarl these intricate reproductive works. Aggressively treating conception-threatening conditions *before* you're ready for a baby is your best insurance against infertility. Here's a list of the chronic conditions you need to get under control *now*.

Diabetes. Type 2 diabetes (also called adult-onset diabetes) is linked to obesity and insulin resistance, both of which can cause hormonal upsets in women, out-of-whack menstrual cycles, and infertility. Chapters 3, 5, and 16 offer solutions for controlling diabetes and insulin resistance.

Type 1 diabetes (sometimes called juvenile-onset or insulin-dependent diabetes) develops when the insulin-producing cells of the pancreas are destroyed by autoantibodies. This process may cause the body to make antibodies that attack other endocrine organs, including the ovaries. The result may be a depletion of eggs and early menopause.

Blood sugar is difficult to control with type 1 diabetes because all of the insulin the body needs must be given by injection. If you do conceive, diabetes can seriously harm your baby if you haven't yet reined in high blood sugar. Women with poorly monitored preexisting diabetes in the early weeks of pregnancy are two to four times more likely to have a baby with birth defects, including neural tube defects like spina bifida. They're also at greater risk of miscarriage, stillbirth, or high-birth-weight babies that are difficult to deliver. If you develop gestational diabetes later in pregnancy, you boost your odds of having a larger-than-normal baby or one with birth defects.

Diabetes affects male fertility as well. Diabetic men often experience retrograde ejaculation, in which semen enters the bladder instead of being ejaculated through the penis into the female reproductive tract where it can fertilize eggs. Diabetes also can cause erectile dysfunction.

High blood pressure. "The relationship between chronic hypertension and infertility isn't clear," notes Kaylen M. Silverberg, M.D., medical director of the Texas Fertility Center in Austin and obstetrics and gynecology professor at the University of Texas Medical Branch in Galveston and the University of Texas Health Science Center at San Antonio. Chronic hypertension does, however, appear to contribute to infertility in certain people (one reason may be the conception-thwarting impact of high blood pressure drugs, which we'll discuss below).

Having uncontrolled high blood pressure while you're pregnant—either because it wasn't under control before conception or because it develops afterward (a condition known as preeclampsia)—can invite serious complications, including constriction of blood vessels in the uterus that cuts off oxygen and nutrients to your baby; separation of the placenta from the uterine wall, which may lead to heavy bleeding and shock; and eclampsia, a life-threatening complication of preeclampsia, which may include convulsions and coma.

Thyroid disease. Having an underactive thyroid gland (hypothyroidism) or an overactive one (hyperthyroidism) can scramble your ovulation cycles and short-circuit your ability to conceive. Hypothyroidism may also be associated with an autoimmune response in your body, signaling it to manufacture antibodies that attack your ovaries and lead to premature menopause.

Autoimmune diseases. Like diabetes and thyroid disease, autoimmune conditions such as lupus (which is accompanied by arthritis-like stiffness and fatigue) also sometimes produce antibodies that attack your body, including your ovaries.

Anemia. While there's no direct link between anemia and infertility, the root causes of anemia occasionally spark fertility problems. "If a woman is anemic because she's malnourished or has an eating disorder, she may have disrupted ovulation," notes Dr. Silverberg. "If she's anemic because of heavy bleeding from a benign fibroid tumor in her uterus, the fibroid may be contributing to her infertility."

CHECK YOUR MEDICINE CABINET

Sometimes it's not a disease that impedes conception, but the treatment. Common medications for everything from acne to ulcers can temporarily foul up your fertility or your partner's.

"It's important to recognize that drugs can affect a whole range of things that cause fertility problems, such as libido, impotence, and depression," notes Dr. Adamson. "Some drugs even affect ovulation and sperm count."

Because drug studies don't always look specifically at fertility, the true reproductive repercussions of many medications aren't known or are based only on animal data. What's more, side effects differ by individual; one person's pain relief may be another's fertility nightmare. As a general rule, Dr. Adamson advises, "Talk to your doctor first about what you and your partner are taking, and if you're trying to get pregnant, always take as few medications as you can."

With your doctor's permission, you may want to toss the following drugs from your medicine cabinet before trying to conceive. If your life depends on any of them, ask your physician about alternatives that are less likely to cut your conception odds.

Drugs That Can Affect Female Fertility

Accutane. An acne treatment containing synthetic vitamin A, Accutane is linked to birth defects, including mental retardation. Because injury can happen in the first few weeks of pregnancy—often before you know you're pregnant—you may want to stop using Accutane or ask your doctor for a safer alternative before trying to conceive.

Antibiotics. By altering cervical mucus patterns, antibiotics sometimes throw off ovulation while you're taking them. Studies have yet to definitively show, however, whether it's the antibiotics that temporarily squelch fertility or the illness being treated.

Antidepressants. Not only can depression drugs scramble your menstrual cycles, temporarily suppressing fertility, but research also indicates that they may boost your baby's risk of birth defects if you use them during pregnancy. For example, monoamine oxidase (MAO) inhibitors such as phenelzine (Nardil) and tranylcypromine (Parnate) have been shown to cause an increased risk of birth defects when taken during the first 3 months of pregnancy. Since you don't always know you're pregnant right away, consider weaning yourself off antidepressants or finding a safer alternative well before you conceive.

Antianxiety drugs. It is unclear how drugs such as diazepam (Valium) and alprazolam (Xanax) affect fertility, but like some antidepressants, their use has been found to cause an increased risk of birth defects during the first trimester. For this reason, it's wise to avoid taking them, if possible, when you're trying to get pregnant.

Cold and flu remedies with antihistamines. Designed to dry up overactive mucous membranes in your nose and throat, these popular remedies also occasionally thicken or dry up cervical mucus. For sperm, that's tantamount to swimming across a bone-dry desert or through a sea of Jell-O. (See chapter 13 for more on cold and cough remedies with expectorants that actually aid swimming sperm by thinning cervical fluids.)

Corticosteroids. Creams and ointments containing corticosteroids are used to relieve the redness, swelling, and itching of skin conditions, like psoriasis. These products can cause irregular menstrual periods, depending on the potency of the drug and the amount used.

High blood pressure medications. Potassium-sparing diuretics that contain spironolactone (such as Aldactone) can also throw off menstrual cycles.

Ibuprofen. Pain relievers, such as Advil or Aleve, sometimes sabotage ovulation, particularly if you take them regularly. "If you're on fertility medication or have been trying unsuccessfully to get pregnant, just stick with acetaminophen (Tylenol)," notes Mitchell N. Essig, M.D., an obstetrics and gynecology instructor at Albert Einstein College of Medicine at Yeshiva University in the Bronx, who also has a private Manhattan practice in reproductive endocrinology and infertility.

Drugs That Can Affect Male Fertility

Anabolic steroids. "Weight lifters use steroids (related to the male sex hormone testosterone) to build muscle," notes Neil Baum, M.D., director of the Impotence Foundation in New Orleans and urology professor at Tulane University School of Medicine in New Orleans and Louisiana State University School of Medicine in Shreveport. "But too much can shut down the pituitary gland and the testicles, causing infertility. Fortunately, most of the time fertility returns within a few weeks after stopping use."

Antidepressants. These libido-altering drugs sometimes lay waste to sexual desire and hinder a man's ability to ejaculate.

Corticosteroids. Men who use these skin preparations for a long time may see a dip in their libidos and sexual abilities.

High blood pressure medications. Potassium-sparing diuretics with spironolactone (such as Aldactone) sometimes blunt sexual desire and interfere with erections. Calcium-channel blockers (including Procardia) may make sperm sluggish, curtailing their ability to penetrate and fertilize eggs. Alpha blockers (like Cardura) can lead to retrograde ejaculation.

Ulcer medications. H_2 blockers with cimetidine (including Tagamet) can impede erections and slow down sperm production.

DON'T GO UNDER THE KNIFE UNNECESSARILY

"It's not as easy as it sounds, but women should really try not to have intra-abdominal or pelvic surgery if they don't need it," notes Dr. Adamson. The reason? Pelvic adhesions. When the body can't heal an injury (caused by surgery or infection) with normal tissue, it employs scar tissue. But scarring inside the pelvic and abdominal cavities can bind organs together, preventing the release of eggs from the ovaries and blocking egg pickup by the fallopian tubes, leading to infertility. In addition, adhesions inside the uterus may wreak havoc with menstrual cycles and are linked to recurrent miscarriages. Men are also at risk for infertility after pelvic trauma or surgery, which can scar reproductive organs, damage nerves required for erection, and obstruct ejaculation of sperm. That's why you and your partner should think twice before having any surgery in your reproductive regions, even if reproductive organs aren't involved. That includes back or hip surgery, an appendectomy, or gall bladder surgery.

Before any procedures, ask your doctor about your chances of getting adhesions and run through any nonsurgical alternatives you might opt for instead. If you aren't getting complete explanations, get a second opinion. If surgery turns out to be your only option, spend the time to find the best and most experienced surgeon. Also, try to avoid multiple surgeries for a single problem; if one surgery doesn't fix your ovarian cyst, for example, another isn't likely to work any better—and could even make things worse.

"Surgery can be very potent, but it doesn't solve every problem every time," Dr. Adamson says. "There's a law of diminishing returns; you don't get as good a result the second, third, or fourth time you try surgical intervention."

The following surgeries can ravage your reproductive system and are often avoidable. Before you go ahead with any of them, weigh the benefits and the risks.

Removal of uterine fibroids. These benign uterine growths are usually symptom-free. Unless they are distorting your uterine cavity or causing heavy bleeding or pain, they can usually be left alone without harm. Removing them may boost your risk of fertility-robbing pelvic and uterine adhesions.

D & C or abortion. During a D & C (dilation and curettage), the cervix is dilated and the uterus emptied. D & Cs are often done to stem excessive uterine bleeding after childbirth and to end pregnancy during the first few days. If the uterus is damaged, though, or an infection develops, uterine adhesions may form.

Abortion is similar to a D & C (the cervix is dilated and a suction tube is inserted into the uterus to remove an unwanted fetus), except it's usually performed between 6 and 12 weeks into a pregnancy. Not only can an abortion spawn uterine adhesions, but it may also cause the fallopian tubes to become infected and scarred, leading to fertility trouble. The more abortions you have (especially three or more), the greater your risk of infertility.

Removal of ovarian cysts. Not all ovarian cysts are created equal. Functional cysts and corpus luteum cysts are usually harmless and go away by themselves after about 3 months. As a general rule, if a cyst is 5 centimeters or larger for more than 3 months or if it's causing extreme pain, you should consider having it removed through surgery or alternative treatments such as transvaginal aspiration. If not, your best bet is to leave it alone.

Removal of adhesions. The good news: If you get adhesions from a previous surgery or infection, you can have them removed, boosting your conception odds. Be forewarned, though, that removing them sometimes backfires, causing more injury—and more adhesions. What's more, adhesions, particularly severe ones, often show up again after surgery.

The bottom line: If you have mild to moderate tubal or ovarian adhesions removed, your likelihood of a full-term pregnancy is between 70 and 80 percent. Your pregnancy odds drop by half if the adhesions are severe.

FIGHT FERTILITY-ROBBING INFECTIONS

Surgery isn't the only thing that scars reproductive organs. Infections are also prime culprits. Even that case of chlamydia you had in your twenties or the urinary tract infection that sent your partner to the doctor last year can inflict lasting reproductive woes (including infertility, pregnancy complications, and birth defects).

The best approach is to avoid infections altogether. Practicing safe sex with condoms, for example, can fend off most fertility-robbing sexually transmitted diseases (STDs).

Because infection dodging isn't always possible, you should get a test for STDs each year when you get your annual gynecological exam and Pap test. You may also want to get tested for some specific infections before you conceive. Chances are your doctor will test for many of the following sexually transmitted infections plus rubella via a simple blood test during your first prenatal visit. But don't count on a test for everything (different states have different requirements).

Because many infections fester for years without symptoms, the earlier you get checked—even months or years before you're ready to get pregnant—the greater your chances of catching something before reproductive harm is permanent. "Many infections can be tested for and treated ahead of time through antibiotics or immunizations so they don't cause problems," says Nancy Green, M.D., medical director of the March of Dimes.

Sexually Transmitted Infections

Chlamydia. Transmitted through unprotected sex with an infected partner, chlamydia infections often smolder undetected for years. In fact, as many as three of every four infected women and 40 percent of infected men don't know they have chlamydia. Unfortunately, discovery often comes after the damage is already done. "Chlamydia is a huge problem," notes Dr. Essig. "It's the most common and most insidious of STDs."

If not treated, chlamydia can lead to fertility-destroying pelvic inflammatory disease (PID), in which harmful bacteria migrate from the urethra and cervix into the upper genital tract, causing infection and scarring in the fallopian tubes. Indeed, one-third to one-half of the one million women who get chlamydia infections each year wind up with PID. Sadly, about 100,000 of these women end up infertile. Women who have been infected with chlamydia are also more prone to tubal, or ectopic, pregnancies, in which fertilized eggs are blocked from reaching the uterus and implant instead in a fallopian tube. Surgery to remove the fetus is not only life-threatening for the mother but also may lead to more scarring.

In men, chlamydia infections also have serious reproductive repercussions, including epididymitis, an inflammation of the epididymis, a series of ducts at the rear of the testicles. If untreated, it may spread to the testes, resulting in infertility.

Gonorrhea. Like chlamydia, the fallout from untreated gonorrhea (half of all cases are symptomless) is sometimes PID; between 10 and 40 percent of women with gonorrhea will develop this serious infection.

In men, gonorrhea can scar the genital tract and keep sperm from being ejaculated.

HIV. The human immunodeficiency virus, which causes AIDS, not only upsets your menstrual cycles but can also infect your baby at birth. Currently, there is no cure for HIV, but if you have it, you can work with your doctor to take steps to prevent it from hurting your unborn child, such as prenatal treatment with HIV-specific medications.

Herpes. "Untreated genital herpes doesn't necessarily cause infertility, but the neurological damage to a baby from exposure at delivery is severe, including cerebral palsy and seizures," says Dr. Essig. That's why being tested and treated beforehand is crucial. If a woman has herpes at the time of delivery, transmission to the baby can usually be avoided if she has a C-section.

Hepatitis B. Like herpes, this virus (usually transmitted sexually or via contact with infected blood) causes liver disease and doesn't necessarily harm fertility. But having an active infection while you're pregnant boosts your chances of passing it on to your baby during delivery. Unfortunately, hepatitis B is often symptomless, so a mom-to-be may not even know she has it.

Most infected people recover and develop an immunity to the virus. If you have chronic hepatitis B infection or fear you might be exposed to the virus during pregnancy, however, consider getting the hepatitis B vaccine. Should you get pregnant shortly after being vaccinated, there's little risk of transmission to your baby because the vaccine contains inactivated (non-infectious) hepatitis B particles. Still, to be safe, think about waiting 3 months after receiving the vaccine to conceive.

Cytomegalovirus (CMV). A member of the herpes family, CMV is usually transmitted sexually or passed on through contact with saliva, urine, blood, or mucus. Those who work in day care centers, nursing homes, and hospitals are usually at greatest risk.

CMV doesn't ordinarily cause symptoms; when symptoms do crop up, they're mostly flulike. Nor is infertility generally an issue. The real worry is that if you're infected during pregnancy or an old infection reactivates (CMV never goes away and can't be cured), you may pass it on to your baby. Most babies born to exposed mothers aren't harmed, but one in seven wind up with neurological problems, including mental retardation and learning disabilities.

If you're at risk for exposure, get tested before trying to conceive. (The virus can be detected through a simple blood test.) If the test shows that you have not had CMV, be careful to avoid high-risk situations before and after conception, advises reproductive endocrinologist and gynecologic surgeon Deborah Metzger, M.D., Ph.D., medical director of Helena Women's Health in San Jose, California, and medical advisor to this book.

Other Infections

Parvovirus. Parvovirus is responsible for a flulike infection called fifth disease. And much like the flu, it's spread via airborne respiratory droplets. Most people have been infected and have developed immunity naturally, but if you get it while you're pregnant, it can attack your baby's blood cells and kill it. Currently, there is no vaccine against it, so it's wise to get tested before conception and take precautions.

Toxoplasmosis. Toxoplasmosis is also called the "litterbox disease." You can easily avoid toxoplasmosis by not eating raw or undercooked meat, which could contain the parasite *Toxoplasma gondii*, and by getting someone else to change your cat's litterbox. Cats who eat infected rodents or birds often pass it on through their feces.

Infertility isn't likely. Nor will you pass toxoplasmosis on to your baby if you had it before getting pregnant and developed an immunity to it. If not—and you have a cat or suspect you're at risk for exposure during pregnancy—you should be tested before trying for a baby and take care while you're pregnant to avoid exposure. Infected babies can develop harmful eye infections, jaundice, and pneumonia. Some even die within a few days of birth.

Urinary tract infections (UTIs). Having a UTI during pregnancy is linked with premature labor and delivery.

Rubella (German measles). Chances are you're immune to rubella, either because you were vaccinated as a child or had the illness. It's wise to be tested before you conceive, however, because you don't always know for sure if you're susceptible and there's a small chance of becoming infected during pregnancy. Rubella can cause mental retardation and blindness in your baby or may lead to miscarriage and stillbirth.

If the blood test shows you don't have rubella antibodies, your doctor will advise you to be vaccinated. The MMR (measles–mumps–rubella) vaccine contains live virus, meaning there's a possibility of infecting your baby with rubella should you become pregnant soon after being vaccinated. Because no studies have shown any rise in birth defects among women who didn't wait to conceive or were vaccinated during pregnancy, however, the Centers for Disease Control and Prevention recently shortened the recommended waiting time between receiving the vaccine and getting pregnant from 3 months to 28 days.

Even so, the jury may still be out on the long-term impact of the MMR vaccine. One recent study suggests that children born to women who received MMR vaccines *after* giving birth tend to have an increased risk for autism disorders. A leading theory is that the live virus might be transmitted through breast milk or directly to the infant, causing later developmental problems. Other studies suggest that children who receive the MMR vaccine after birth also exhibit more autism disorders. Your best bet: If you need an MMR vaccine, get it as far in advance of conception as possible.

Chickenpox. Like rubella, if you've already had chickenpox, don't worry about passing it on to your baby. If you've never had it, however, think about getting tested and vaccinated before conception. Keep in mind, though, that only about 2 percent of babies whose mothers are infected while carrying them are born with birth defects, which can include seizures and mental retardation. If your risk of exposure is high and you opt for the vaccine, medical experts recommend waiting 1 month after receiving it before trying to conceive.

PRESERVE FERTILITY AFTER CANCER TREATMENT

After Lindsay Nohr received a second diagnosis of tongue cancer at age 24, her oncologist pushed her immediately into an aggressive round of radiation therapy, chemotherapy, and surgery. She was concerned about the impact on her fertility, but doctors told her not to worry because Lance Armstrong, the champion bicyclist, had fathered a child after undergoing similar treatment for testicular cancer.

"That's when I panicked," she recalls. "I knew that Armstrong's treatment had made him sterile and the only reason he had children is because he froze his sperm ahead of time."

Determined not to miss out on motherhood, Nohr plunged into researching her options. But it was tough going. Many doctors she spoke to either didn't know much about safeguarding fertility or were so anxious to start treatment right away that they didn't want to wait while she took steps to protect herself.

"Most oncologists are so focused on survival that they don't think about quality-of-life issues, like fertility," says Roger G. Gosden, D.Sc., Ph.D., scientific director of the Jones Institute for Reproductive Medicine at Eastern Virginia Medical School in Norfolk and professor of obstetrics and gynecology. As a result, many patients never know—until it's too late—that the very treatments needed to save their lives might also render them sterile.

For men, any cancer treatment, including removing tumors from reproductive organs and undergoing radiation and chemotherapy (which destroys both healthy and unhealthy cells throughout the entire body), can permanently destroy the ability to produce or ejaculate sperm.

Women, in turn, face two hurdles. If cancer treatment doesn't leave them sterile, they may go through early menopause (premature ovarian failure, or POF) later on. Reports suggest that women undergoing chemotherapy or radiation during their reproductive years increase their risk of infertility by 40 percent to 80 percent, and more than two-thirds eventually experience POF. (The risk of premature menopause is directly related to the age of the woman and the type of chemotherapy she receives. Furthermore, it may take 18 months or longer for periods to resume after chemotherapy.)

The good news is that many fertility-preserving options are now available, and more are on the way. Nohr ultimately chose to freeze her unfertilized eggs (see the section on oocyte cryopreservation). Before she began chemotherapy, doctors retrieved 29 eggs from her ovaries. The eggs are now in deep freeze at Stanford Medical Center until she's married and knows for sure whether she's infertile. If so, she plans to have the eggs fertilized by her future husband's sperm and implanted in her uterus via in vitro fertilization (IVF).

"I don't want to become infertile, but chances are I will," says Nohr, who has since started a Web site for other cancer survivors hoping to preserve their fertility (www.fertilehope.org). "Now I have a backup plan—extra insurance."

If you or your partner is facing cancer treatment and worried about infertility, here are some options to consider.

Options for Women

Embryo cryopreservation. If a woman has a partner or is willing to accept sperm from a donor, she can have mature or immature eggs removed from her ovaries, fertilized via standard IVF, and frozen for later implantation in her uterus.

Embryo freezing has a good success rate—for every three embryos, there's about a 40 percent chance of successful pregnancy if you're under 35. Success rates are lower for older women. The downside, though, is that it can take 4 to 5 weeks to finish the necessary rounds of ovary-stimulating hormones and harvest eggs. If you need chemotherapy right away, you may not have the luxury of time. Nor can everyone afford it (many insurers won't pay for embryo cryopreservation). The average cost per IVF cycle is $10,000, plus $350 a year for embryo storage.

Oocyte (unfertilized egg) cryopreservation. If you don't have a partner or don't want a sperm donor, you can freeze your unfertilized eggs, like Nohr, until you're ready for pregnancy. At that point, eggs are thawed, fertilized, and implanted in your uterus. The cost is slightly lower than that for embryo freezing (about $8,000 per IVF cycle, plus $350 a year for storage), but the procedure is still relatively new and eggs are less likely to survive freezing than embryos. Those that do have about a 3 to 6 percent chance of successful fertilization into embryos that result in full-term pregnancy.

Ovarian tissue cryopreservation. Although this procedure is still experimental, the idea behind it is to preserve ovarian tissue and the thousands of immature eggs it contains. That way, you have many more eggs to work with when you're ready for pregnancy. Although study results are encouraging, the biggest problem so far has been storing ovarian tissue and transplanting it back into the body without damaging it.

There are several ways to do this. The easiest is to remove one ovary, cut it into strips, and freeze them. The strips are later transplanted back into the pelvis or arm, and the woman is given ovary-stimulating hormones to produce eggs, which are then fertilized and implanted in the uterus. The procedure works in animals and looks promising for humans, although so far no babies have been born using it.

Another method is to freeze the entire ovary, then transplant it back in place later on for egg harvesting. "It's been difficult to store the whole organ because of ice crystal damage during the cooling process," notes Dr. Gosden. "But the procedure has now been done with rats and could be done in humans one day."

Ultimately, doctors will be able to grow ovarian tissue outside the body, harvest eggs, and implant them via IVF. "This avoids the risk of returning ovarian tissue to a patient who's not in full remission or still has lingering effects of treatment," Dr. Gosden notes.

Gonadotropin-releasing hormone (GnRH) analogue. Girls who haven't yet reached puberty tend to have higher fertility rates after undergoing chemotherapy than women whose reproductive organs are already mature. GnRH analogue is a hormone-blocking agent that is given in conjunction with chemotherapy to temporarily throw the reproductive system into a state of prepubescence (akin to temporary menopause) and hopefully maintain fertility.

So far, studies of this highly experimental procedure have yielded mixed results in humans; in some cases, ovarian function has returned, but no one is sure if it's the GnRH at work or other factors. If the procedure does ultimately prove effective, GnRH may be a good choice for cancer patients who don't have time to wait for retrieval of eggs or ovarian tissue.

Oophoropexy. A fairly simple procedure, oophoropexy involves temporarily tying the ovaries out of the way of radiation (often behind the uterus) so they aren't exposed to fertility-destroying doses. The only drawback, notes Dr. Gosden, is that it works only for patients undergoing radiation, not chemotherapy.

Radical trachelectomy. In lieu of a fertility-robbing hysterectomy, women with early cervical cancer can opt to have only the malignant part of their cervix removed, leaving the uterus intact. Although still a new procedure, radical trachelectomy has proven successful in a number of women.

Options for Men

Sperm banking. Before undergoing chemotherapy or radiation, a man can freeze sperm for safekeeping until he's ready to start a family. At that time, sperm can be placed in his partner's uterus for natural fertilization to occur.

Success depends largely on sperm quality (cancer can impair and weaken sperm). Thus, the more donations a man makes, the better his chances of banking enough hardy sperm to achieve later fertilization and pregnancy. With newer techniques like intracytoplasmic sperm injection, in which a single sperm is injected directly into an egg rather than undergoing the normal fertilization route, only one viable sperm is now actually needed.

Testicular tissue preservation. Sperm banking is almost always offered to

WHAT WORKED FOR US

SHE PRESERVED HER FERTILITY WHILE BEATING CANCER

At 18, when most people are heading off to college or setting out on their own, Tara Heiskell received devastating news: She had stage 3 Hodgkin's disease. Her best chance of beating it was a grueling combination of chemotherapy and radiation, but treatment also carried a steep price. If chemotherapy didn't destroy her fertility, doctors warned, radiation to her groin almost certainly would.

"I went through with chemo because I didn't really think it would affect my fertility," she remembers. "But when it came time for radiation, my first reaction was, 'Forget it.' I knew I eventually wanted to get married and have children and figured I'd take my chances at not having treatment."

Horrified, her doctors cautioned that forgoing radiation meant almost certain death. But Tara stood firm. Not long afterward, her radiation oncologist handed her an article about a procedure called an oophoropexy, in which the ovaries are tied behind the uterus for protection during radiation. Although the procedure had been performed only a few times, Tara decided it was her best shot at both staying alive and becoming a mother.

She and her surgeon consulted with a fertility specialist familiar with the procedure. Days later, a team of doctors placed a laparoscope through a small incision in her belly button and made two tiny incisions through which specialized instruments were used to tie her ovaries behind her uterus. A special suture designed to dissolve in 6 to 8 weeks was used so that Tara's ovaries would drop back in place without more surgery once the radiation was completed. "Doctors were pretty certain it would work," she says. But only time would tell for sure.

One month later, in July 1992, Tara met the man who would one day become her husband. Their first son was born in 1995, and the couple had a second son in 1998. Both of Tara's pregnancies progressed normally and free of problems.

"Thanks to the fact that I knew to ask questions and push the issue and had caring, knowledgeable doctors who wanted to help, my fertility was saved," says Tara. The mother of two has now been free of Hodgkin's disease for almost 10 years.

men who have no children or are under 55, Dr. Gosden notes, but it doesn't work for boys who aren't yet producing sperm and men who don't have good sperm specimens because they're older or because illness has affected their sperm quality. For these men and boys, hope is on the horizon. Testicular tissue preservation is still in the experimental stage, but the idea is to surgically remove testicular tissue, which contains immature sperm, freeze it, and then inject fledgling sperm back into the testes when pregnancy is desired. The procedure is similar to ovarian tissue cryopreservation, which involves removing ovarian tissue with its undeveloped eggs. So far, testicular tissue preservation appears to work in animals, and preliminary human studies are "encouraging," Dr. Gosden says.

PART THREE

THE GET-PREGNANT-NOW PLAN

11

The Power of Preconception Care

You and your husband fantasize about what another human being would look like who would share your features. Families playing at the park have become more interesting than a Hollywood drama. You begin to melt over the cherub-faced toddlers captured in photographs you never before noticed on your coworkers' desks. There's a cosmic pull of sorts that lures you out of the misses section and into the miniature fuzzy jumper section of your favorite department store.

If you both agree you've evolved from hoping to have a child "someday" to wanting to take the big leap, it's time to make some serious plans. That doesn't mean booking a sultry penthouse for the weekend, tossing your birth control pills, and brainstorming baby names. It's not the most romantic advice, but experts strongly recommend stepping back and taking time to evaluate your pregnancy readiness. By making sure both you and your partner are in the best possible health before you try to have a child, you not only can increase your chances of conceiving but can also prevent health complications to both you and your baby down the road.

In earlier chapters, you read about general preconception guidelines in the areas of nutrition, proper weight range, fitness, resolving bad habits, contraception, emotional health, and avoiding toxins. Now is the time to catch up with any of these goals you haven't yet accomplished. It's also the time to schedule a visit with your gynecologist, family doctor, nurse-midwife, or nurse-practitioner so that you can identify any other areas of preconception care that you might need, advises the American College of Obstetricians and Gynecologists.

For example, women 35 and older are twice as likely to develop high blood pressure or diabetes during pregnancy than are younger mothers. But women who take steps to enhance their health before conceiving can significantly reduce their risks for these complications. "Preconception care is not a luxury," says Nancy Green, M.D. As the medical director of the March of Dimes, Dr. Green is acutely aware of the difficult pregnancies and childhood illnesses associated with poor pregnancy planning. The March of Dimes estimates that 30 to 40 percent of birth defects are caused by medical, environmental, genetic, and psychosocial factors that could, to some degree, be prevented.

"Preconception care is a window of opportunity to optimize both partners' health and identify any risks and take the steps to reduce them," explains Dr. Green. Even the healthiest young couple should expect to heighten their level of self-care and physical readiness in the months before first trying to conceive.

PARTNER WITH YOUR PRACTITIONERS

Not communicating your conception plans to your health care practitioners is like a parachuter jumping out of an airplane and *then* considering an equipment safety check. Even your dentist has special considerations if you are thinking of conceiving. (She may want to push up or delay a procedure to prevent exposing a fetus to anesthesia.) Furthermore, women 35 and older are advised to get their baseline or annual mammogram done before conception, since pregnancy and lactation may delay your next screening.

Your first order of business is to work with your physician to get chronic health conditions under control. Diabetes, high blood pressure, seizures, kidney disease, systemic lupus erythematosus, and phenylke-tonuria all carry well-known risks to mother and baby. You and your doctor will need to make special efforts to stabilize these conditions and adjust medications to pregnancy-safe doses.

In addition to catching up with all your standard medical care, your preconception visit should include a routine set of questions and tests for a couple preparing for pregnancy. Ideally, you should schedule the appointment for 6 months before you begin trying to conceive. "However, not every medical practice is accustomed to a special preconception visit," points out Lisa Summers, C.N.M., Dr.Ph., a public health expert and spokesperson for the American College of Nurse-Midwives in Washington, D.C. Be aware that your doctor may not routinely offer preconception care and that your insurance company will probably not cover the visit. "Insurance companies erroneously consider prenatal care and preconception care two separate codes. We're working to change that," Dr. Summers adds.

Standard preconception visits usually include the following evaluations. If your doctor doesn't traditionally provide preconception appointments, you may need to request these services individually.

* A complete physical. Your doctor should be up to date on your complete family health history, including first-, second-, and third-degree relatives who died early or have chronic health problems, birth defects, or known genetic diseases. This information may lead to a referral to a genetics counselor. Make sure you also discuss all medications, herbs, and nutritional supplements you are taking, since they may need to be modified for pregnancy. Be sure to ask your practitioner if your weight is within 15 percent of your ideal body mass index; if it's not, you may need to alter your exercise program and diet, adds Alan Copperman, M.D., assistant professor of obstetrics, gynecology, and reproductive medicine at Mount Sinai Medical Center in New York City.

* Blood and urine tests. These tests should determine whether you have diabetes and identify any nutritional deficiencies, such as anemia.

Your practitioner may refer you to a nutritionist to correct nutritional deficiencies. Even if your nutrition levels are adequate, all women considering pregnancy are still advised to start taking 400 micrograms of folic acid as soon as possible, says Dr. Green.

* Testing for immunological concerns. Your blood tests should check for exposure to rubella and toxoplasmosis. If you have not been exposed, you can protect your baby from rubella by undergoing immunization; to protect him against toxoplasmosis, you'll need to simply take extra precautions to avoid exposure. You should also be screened for hepatitis B, hepatitis C, HIV, or tuberculosis if you are at risk for exposure to any of these diseases (from foreign travel or working in a health care profession, for example). Together, you and your doctor can decide if you should be immunized for these or any other illnesses, such as chickenpox, Lyme disease, and tetanus. If you're vaccinated with a killed or attenuated virus, you'll need to wait 1 to 3 months before trying to conceive to prevent exposing an active virus to a fetus.

* A complete gynecological exam. A key component of preconception care is a standard pelvic exam, Pap test, and cervical cultures for chlamydia, gonorrhea, mycoplasma, and ureaplasma. You and your practitioner can develop a plan to phase out contraception when all your preconception screenings and interventions are complete. If you haven't yet discussed your complete menstrual, reproductive, and contraceptive history, now is the time. In addition, you and your partner will need an infertility workup if you've never resolved the cause of recurrent miscarriages or delayed fertility. If you have a history of using intrauterine devices, your doctor may need to do additional tests to see if your fallopian tubes are open.

* Screening for sexually transmitted diseases. Your physician will ask you for a history of any genital symptoms you've experienced that may indicate a need for testing. Testing both partners for chlamydia, gonorrhea, syphilis, and HIV is becoming part of standard preconception

care. Remember that although you may not have symptoms of any of these conditions, they may endanger the life of an unborn child and your reproductive future.

* Substance abuse intervention. The bottom line is that no amount of alcohol, tobacco, caffeine, or illegal drugs has been proven safe to use during pregnancy. It is imperative that you are "clean" before you try to conceive.

* A discussion of your mental readiness. Be open with your practitioners about the help you need regarding relationship problems as well as other inhibitions or fears related to childbearing, advises Dr. Summers. Stress can actually prevent you from ovulating on schedule, so getting help for problems that are troubling you—whether they're related to work, your relationship with your partner or family, or even your self-esteem—should be a priority.

Be sure to let your practitioner know if you are prone to depression or if you experienced postpartum depression with a previous pregnancy. If necessary, your doctor may refer you to a mental health professional so that you can address any mental health issues before conception.

Mental preparation also includes working out a plan for maternity leave from work as well as financial coverage of maternity expenses. After you have your child, will you stay at home or return to work? What about child care? (Keep in mind that for some day care centers, you need to get your name on the waiting list as soon as you find out you're pregnant.) What kind of family support can you expect? Clarity about these issues is a necessary form of stress control, among other benefits.

GENETIC COUNSELING

Genetic specialists are commonly thought of as the people who perform amniocentesis, chorionic villus sampling (CVS), and other strange-sounding tests on "high-risk" babies in the womb. But there are numerous reasons to become acquainted with genetic specialists while you are still thinking of conceiving.

First, you'll need a quick primer on the roles of the various genetic spe-

FERTILITYVISIONARIES

Belinda Barnes and the Foresight Program

Foresight: The Association for the Promotion of Preconceptual Care was established in 1978 by Belinda Barnes, a British nursery nurse. Her original mission was to decrease the rates of childhood problems such as attention deficit hyperactivity disorder (ADHD), allergies, birth defects, and learning disabilities, which are linked to poor nutrition and other adverse conditions in the preconception and pregnancy stages. She discovered the program also worked to improve the odds of couples who were unable to conceive until they made health and lifestyle changes.

Barnes organized a medical advisory board consisting of family doctors, alternative health practitioners, and nutritionists to research and develop a comprehensive preconception program. This program is designed to give couples a healthier start and to offer affordable, safe solutions to those with a history of miscarriage, stillbirth, birth defects, unexplained infertility, postnatal depression, and other complications of pregnancy and birth.

Foresight has become the gold standard for preconception care in the United Kingdom. In fact, Foresight's success rates have been nothing short of amazing. Researchers at Surrey University tracked a random 367 British couples enrolled in the Foresight Program in 1990 who varied in age and health status. Not only did 89 percent of the total group conceive, but 86 percent of the 204 couples *who were previously infertile* conceived. In fact, according to written and telephone follow-up surveys conducted in 1993, not a single participant in the Foresight program experienced miscarriage, stillbirth, malformation, or an unhealthy infant—even those with prior histories.

Surrey researchers forecasted that an identical cross section of British couples not following Foresight guidelines would experience more than 92 miscarriages, 11 malformations, and 5 stillbirths. When it comes to overcoming infertility,

cialists. *Genetic counselors* are generally nonphysicians who assess the likelihood of a genetic problem before or after conception and determine what type of testing is necessary. If a problem is found, the counselor will advise you on the probability of having a healthy child and what may be done to

participants in U.S. assisted-reproduction programs have far less success (with an average of 24 percent live births).

Couples enrolled in the Foresight program complete thorough questionnaires assessing their medical history and lifestyle. Men and women are given a hair analysis that can help detect heavy-metal contaminants and trace mineral deficiencies. Nutritionists advise on a "whole food" diet with no refined carbohydrates and plenty of fresh, raw foods, such as fruit and salads, and high-quality protein. Where indicated by the history, they will also look for hidden allergies, nutritional imbalances, and intestinal parasites. In addition, couples are screened for genitourinary infections at the nearest hospital. The men get their prostatic secretions evaluated for any hidden infection, along with semen analysis and blood and urine tests.

Six months are reserved for correcting any problems, while couples take specially developed Foresight nutritional supplements (as indicated by the hair analyses) and are educated on essentials like ovulation timing and the dangers of alcohol, smoking, street drugs, and many other environmental hazards. Counselors discuss everything from how to lessen electromagnetic exposure in the home to the best kind of cookware to use for all the organic produce they encourage their clients to eat.

Contact information: More than 140 clinics in the United Kingdom offer the Foresight program, and there are overseas branches in the United States, Australia, and South Africa. To receive an information packet and the location of the nearest Foresight practitioner in your area, send a letter of interest and a self-addressed envelope to Foresight, 28 The Paddock, Godalming, Surrey, England GU7 1XD. You can reach their switchboard by calling 011-44-1483-427839 or log on to www.foresight-preconception.org.uk for more information.

minimize the risk of genetic problems. *Geneticists* are either M.D.'s or Ph.D.'s who do research in genetics or who may see patients who are affected by genetic diseases. *High-risk obstetricians* perform CVS or amniocentesis and specialize in the care of women with high-risk pregnancies. Finally, *pediatric surgeons* may operate on babies in the womb or perform testing on them.

Be aware that certain ethnic backgrounds increase the likelihood of inheritable diseases, such as Tay-Sachs in people of Eastern European Jewish ancestry, sickle-cell anemia in Latino and Black persons, cystic fibrosis in Whites, and thalassemia in people of Mediterranean, African, and Southern Asian descent.

Outside of ethnicity, you may simply have a higher incidence of mental retardation in your family as carriers of the Fragile X gene. Recent technology makes it possible to run a simple blood test that determines whether parents are carriers of these birth defects. The test's ability to ease your mind with the reassurance that you don't actually carry a hereditary illness is priceless.

Other categories of inheritable health problems may include certain forms of cancer, lung diseases, and neurological or neuromuscular diseases such as muscular dystrophy. If there is a history of any of these diseases in your family, genetic counseling may be warranted. If couples are confirmed as carriers, they may wish to conceive differently than they originally planned. While in vitro fertilization isn't for everyone, it sometimes is an option to prevent passing a disease on to a child, notes Dr. Copperman. By consulting with a genetic counselor, you at least can make a well-informed decision about whether or not this option is right for you.

Finally, some couples discover that they are carriers of a disease during early genetic counseling, and it affects their decision concerning whether or not to have a baby, says Dr. Copperman. If this is your situation, you and your partner might want to make the difficult decision to forgo a pregnancy altogether.

Not all inheritable conditions can be diagnosed in advance, however.

Women in the 35-and-older age bracket, for instance, may be referred to genetic specialists for a general discussion of the statistically higher rate of chromosomal disorders associated with older eggs and sperm. The benefit of educating yourself and your partner about this possibility during the preconception stage is that you can choose to buy more time in order to emotionally, mentally, and financially prepare for the additional requirements of a child who may be mentally or physically challenged, Dr. Green points out. Once the pregnancy is under way, a couple can then make early, informed arrangements with their genetic specialists for aggressive prenatal care—such as those amniocentesis and CVS tests the geneticists are so famous for.

12

Master Ovulation Awareness

The conventional wisdom about female fertility is that a woman is most likely to get pregnant around the time she ovulates—usually day 14 of an average 28-day menstrual cycle.

Too bad the conventional wisdom is seldom true.

It's a rare woman whose menstrual cycle is exactly 28 days long; most women have cycles that fall within an average range of 24 to 36 days. In fact, at any given time, nearly 75 percent of women will enter their "fertile window" before day 10 or after day 17, says Toni Weschler, M.P.H., who has developed the Fertility Awareness Method of ovulation detection and is the author of *Taking Charge of Your Fertility*. And even if your period is as predictable as the sunrise, you may not always release an egg: Outside factors such as stress, illness, too much exercise, and interrupted sleep can disrupt ovulation.

Given that we often ovulate before or after we're "supposed" to (and sometimes not at all), it's crucial that women who want to get pregnant learn to recognize—and act on—the subtle and not-so-subtle physical signs that they're ripe to conceive. Unfortunately, few of us were taught to recognize these signs. This lack of knowledge has resulted in countless unnecessary visits to fertility clinics, says Joseph B. Stanford, M.D., associate professor of family and preventive medicine at the University of Utah School of Medicine in Salt Lake City. But here's the encouraging news: Dr. Stanford notes that perhaps about 20 percent of couples who have trouble conceiving aren't infertile at all—they're simply timing intercourse incorrectly. And if you're over 35 and have no cause for infertility other than age, he says, you're as likely to get pregnant using well-timed lovemaking as you are using in vitro fertilization—at considerable cost savings. (And, hopefully, more pleasure.)

Fertility awareness methods don't just up your odds of conceiving, says Victoria H. Jennings, Ph.D., director of the Institute for Reproductive Health at Georgetown University School of Medicine in Washington, D.C. Couples who've used them report that the experience drew them closer, she notes. And as women become more adept at reading their bodies, they tend to feel a new sense of pride in their femininity. It's empowering for women to know about fertility awareness methods, says Dr. Jennings. "When they learn about them, the typical reaction is, 'Why didn't anyone tell me about this before?'" she says.

Here's the beautiful part: Dr. Stanford says that pinpointing your most fertile days is simple, once you understand the workings of your cycle and recognize the clues each stage provides. Consulting an instructor trained in fertility awareness methods can be helpful in learning how the clues work in your own body, he advises.

YOUR BODY'S FERTILITY CLUES

As discussed in chapter 2, a woman's menstrual cycle is synchronized by various hormones, which are released at precise moments and in particular amounts. Each hormone helps ready your body for possible pregnancy and triggers physical "fertility clues." Monitoring these clues can help you home in on the days you're most likely to conceive.

After your period ends each month, your levels of the female sex hormone estrogen gradually rise, and up to 20 egg-containing follicles begin to mature in your ovaries. Only one (the most mature) or occasionally two of these eggs will be released and possibly fertilized. As ovulation approaches, your cervix softens, opens, and pulls up higher. It also begins to manufacture clear, stringy mucus that allows sperm to enter the uterus and fallopian tubes. These are fertility clues one and two.

Near midcycle, the pituitary gland releases luteinizing hormone (LH), which triggers the largest egg to burst through the ovarian wall and begin its journey through the fallopian tube. Once there, the egg will either disintegrate within 24 hours or be fertilized and implanted in the uterus. The follicle that held the egg, called the corpus luteum, remains in the ovary and begins to produce progesterone. In response to this rise in progesterone, your basal body temperature rises nearly one degree and remains higher until your next period. Voilà: fertility clue three. After ovulation, your cervix drops, closes, and grows firmer. Your cervical mucus dries, forming a plug that keeps sperm out until you ovulate again.

In 1 year, a woman with normal fertility who's having regular intercourse has about an 85 percent chance of getting pregnant, says Dr. Jennings. But unless a woman monitors her fertility clues, her chances of conceiving in any given cycle are only about 25 to 30 percent, Dr. Jennings notes. That's because sperm can live only 5 to 6 days and an egg no more than 24 hours after ovulation. So your actual "fertility window" is only about 6 days per cycle, including the 5 days before ovulation and the day of ovulation.

Your chances of conceiving, however, aren't equally high on all 6 days. "A sperm has a better chance of success if it is ready and waiting in the reproductive tract when the egg begins moving down the fallopian tube at ovulation," says Dr. Jennings. Translation: A sperm that's had the chance to swim up your reproductive tract after Monday-night lovemaking has a better chance of meeting up with your egg during ovulation on Wednesday than does a sperm just beginning its journey on Wednesday. Indeed, these early-bird sperm have a 25 to almost 35 percent chance of finding their way to your egg in the 2 days prior to ovulation. After that, the odds drop precipitously, says Dr. Jennings.

WHAT WORKED FOR US

CONCEPTION WAS ALL IN THE TIMING FOR THIS COUPLE

Three years ago, after months of trying to conceive, Julie Lovisa and her husband, Keith, were facing the disturbing possibility that they might be infertile. Then, at a local bookstore, Julie stumbled upon *Taking Charge of Your Fertility*, written by Toni Weschler, M.P.H, developer of the Fertility Awareness Method of ovulation detection.

What she read changed her life—and her approach to getting pregnant.

Using Weschler's method, Julie began monitoring changes in her cervical mucus and charting her basal body temperature every day. It soon became clear that she and Keith had been timing lovemaking all wrong. "I'd just assumed that day 14 was my peak time," she recalls. "But it turned out that I don't ovulate until day 18 or 19. It's amazing what I didn't know about my body."

Julie also discovered that her luteal phase (the number of days after ovulation until menstruation starts) was only 9 days long—potentially too short for implantation of a fertilized egg. She and Keith started timing intercourse to coincide with her later ovulation. Within 2 months, she was pregnant with their daughter and easily conceived her son 2 years later using the same approach.

"We're done having children, but I still use fertility awareness just to see where I am in my cycle and when I'll get my period," says Julie. "I'm also thinking of using it as a contraceptive because I'm almost 35 and have high blood pressure, so I can't be on the Pill."

YOUR FERTILITY AWARENESS OPTIONS

Here's a rundown of the most common fertility prediction methods. Understand, though, that it's not yet known which method best predicts your most fertile days, or which helps a woman conceive most quickly, says Dr. Stanford. His research suggests, however, that methods that pinpoint the 6-day fertile window leading up to and including ovulation are more likely to result in pregnancy. For this reason, they're listed first. But remember: The approach that's right for you and your partner is the one that you're most comfortable with.

Cervical mucus. With this method, you check the consistency of your cervical mucus daily starting the day after your period ends. You then record your observations on a special chart. (Later in this chapter, we provide a chart that you can use.) According to Dr. Stanford's research, this method may be all you need to pinpoint your most fertile days. And even if you have irregular cycles, your secretions should follow a predictable pattern that helps you peg your best preovulatory baby-making days, he says.

"CONGRATULATIONS! IT'S A . . ."

Humans have long tried to influence the sex of their offspring—often by employing the most unusual means. In ancient Greece, women who wanted a boy lay on their right side while they made love and on their left if they longed for a girl. In the Middle Ages, couples drank a mixture of lion's blood and wine, then made love under a full moon to conceive a boy. And in 1916, W. Wallace Hoffman, M.D., published a book that advised parents to "think" their way to the boy or girl of their choice.

Not surprisingly, these approaches have gone by the wayside. But the desire to predetermine a baby's sex has never dimmed. Witness the ongoing success of the 1970 super-seller *How to Choose the Sex of Your Baby*, by Landrum B. Shettles, M.D., Ph.D., and David M. Rorvik. In his book, Dr. Shettles theorizes that intercourse timed close to ovulation, when cervical secretions are most alkaline and favorable to fertilization, favors boys because male sperm are faster and smaller and, under these ideal conditions, are likelier to reach an egg first. Intercourse timed a day or two *before* ovulation, when cervical secretions are still somewhat acidic, theoretically favors slower but hardier female sperm, which arrive to claim the prize—the egg—after male sperm have languished in the inhospitable mucus.

Thousands of satisfied couples swear by the Shettles Method, which boasts a 75 percent or better success rate. But most studies that have examined the method suggest that timing techniques don't work any better than lion's blood and wine. "If you want to try it for fun, okay," says Joseph B. Stanford, M.D., associate professor of family practice at the University of Utah School of Medicine in Salt Lake City. "But don't count on it."

The first few days after your period ends, your vagina will probably feel moist but will not secrete mucus. Over the next few days, or later on in long cycles, you'll observe secretions that are thick, cloudy, sticky, and whitish or yellowish. You should consider these days fertile.

As ovulation approaches, secretions become clearer, more abundant, and slippery, and they may stretch 2 or more inches between your thumb and forefinger. This sperm-friendly mucus resembles your partner's seminal fluid in that it provides a temporary alkaline environment in the normally acidic vagina. It's your body's way of ensuring that sperm are protected and mobile at the time you're most fertile. This is the best time for intercourse. Make love either every day or every other day until after the peak or last day of this fertile-quality mucus. After that, says Dr. Stanford, secretions grow thick and cloudy again or disappear until after your next period.

Perhaps the best-known mucus-monitoring approach is the Billings Ovulation Method. This method was developed in the 1960s by Evelyn Billings, M.D., an Australian pediatrician, and her husband, John Billings, M.D., a neurologist. To learn more or to find a practitioner, check out the Billings Ovulation Method Association—USA Web site at www. boma-usa.org, visit www.billingsmethod.com, or read the book *The Billings Method: Controlling Fertility without Drugs and Devices.*

The Creighton Model FertilityCare System, a standardized variation on the Billings method, uses a scientifically tested scoring system to rate the quality of cervical mucus rather than just its consistency. The method is known for the rigorous professional training it provides to teachers and the standardized instruction procedures it offers couples. Frequent follow-up and support is standard during the first year. Check out the American Academy of FertilityCare Professionals' Web site at www.aafcp.org, or visit www.creightonmodel.com for the name of a certified doctor or teacher.

If you're willing to take classes, consider using either the Creighton or Billings approach, recommends Dr. Stanford. Studies suggest that among couples without fertility problems, those who use either approach may conceive faster than those who don't. (Infertile couples weren't studied.) In

FERTILITY AWARENESS METHODS: FOUR THINGS YOU MUST KNOW

Thinking of trying one or more of the fertility awareness methods in this chapter? Keep the following in mind.

* Because a woman's cycles can fluctuate from month to month, most fertility awareness methods pad the 6-day fertility window with a few extra days. For a more precise calculation of your super-fertile days, consider learning the ropes from an instructor certified by a natural family planning teacher training program. A local family planning or Planned Parenthood clinic can help you find one.

* If you're over 35 and trying to conceive, use these methods for 6 months, tops (1 year, tops, if you're under 35). If you don't get pregnant within these time frames, consult a doctor.

* Think you can't use these methods because your cycles aren't regular? Not so, says Toni Weschler, M.P.H., developer of the Fertility Awareness Method of ovulation detection and author of *Taking Charge of Your Fertility*. With practice, even women with irregular cycles can learn to chart them, she says. Besides, you may not be "irregular" at all. Your body may simply follow its own cycle, ovulating every 35 days, say, instead of every 28.

* Conditions that can cause infertility, such as polycystic ovary syndrome (PCOS), or infertility treatments (including clomiphene citrate [Clomid]) can disrupt or mask a woman's fertility signs, says Weschler. If either is a concern for you, she recommends that you talk to your doctor about the possibility of teaming fertility awareness approaches with your treatment.

one study, more than three-quarters of couples who used the Creighton method conceived in the first month, and the rest had conceived by the seventh month. In a different study, it took 6 months for three-quarters of couples not charting fertility to conceive, and after a year, 1 in 10 still weren't pregnant.

If you want a simpler approach, try the TwoDay Method. Dr. Jennings and her colleagues ran a statistical analysis of thousands of cervical mucus charts and found that it's not necessarily the *type* of mucus that's important in determining fertility but merely the *presence* of mucus. Very simply, if you notice secretions on the current or previous day, then you're probably fertile. No secretions on either day means you're probably not. Check out the Institute for Reproductive Health's Web site at www.irh.org for more information.

Basal body (resting) temperature (BBT). In a normal cycle, a woman's temperature rises almost one degree just after ovulation and remains higher through the beginning of her next cycle. With the BBT method, you take your temperature first thing each morning with a special thermometer

TAKE *HIS* TEMPERATURE, TOO

If you decide to use the basal body (resting) temperature (BBT) method either alone or with another approach, take your partner's temperature along with your own. This little tip helped Erica Frank, M.D., professor in the department of family and preventive medicine at Emory University School of Medicine in Atlanta, Georgia, conceive her child—and it may help you, too.

Dr. Frank came up with this brainstorm after her own frustrating attempts to get pregnant using BBT. "As any woman who has used this method knows, outside influences (like room temperature and the amount of blankets on the bed) can affect your temperature," she says. "I thought, 'Wouldn't it be nice if I could compare my temperature to someone else's—someone who wasn't ovulating?' That's when I decided to use my husband."

Each morning immediately upon awakening, Dr. Frank took her temperature, then her husband's. After 5 months, she found that their temperatures were virtually identical—until she ovulated. Then, hers rose, indicating that she'd ovulated, while his stayed normal.

Dr. Frank—who credits this method with helping her conceive her son, Nathaniel Etheridge—subsequently tested her new-and-improved BBT method on 12 other couples, with similar results. The resulting study was published in the prestigious medical journal *Obstetrics & Gynecology.* "We were very excited about publishing our method," says Dr. Frank. "It was clear to us that it could help other couples conceive, as we believed it had helped us."

known as a basal body thermometer. (You can purchase one in most drug-stores.) It's important to take your temperature before you even get out of bed—no brushing your teeth or inserting contact lenses—because movement affects body temperature. When your temperature spikes, you'll know you have ovulated.

But using basal body temperature alone isn't your best option, says Dr. Stanford, because it can't detect those peak fertility days *before* ovulation. (Recall that once ovulation occurs, conception is less likely, because an egg lives only a few hours and sperm need time to migrate up your reproductive tract.)

If your temperature doesn't rise, you're not ovulating, which makes BBT a good way to identify a potential fertility problem, says Weschler. While anovulatory cycles may be due to a temporary problem like stress or illness, they can also be caused by a more serious problem, including polycystic ovary syndrome, also known as Stein–Leventhal disease, which can cause infertility. See your doctor if you suspect you're not ovulating.

In addition, if you notice more than one temperature spike per month, notify your doctor, advises reproductive endocrinologist and gynecologic surgeon Deborah Metzger, M.D., Ph.D., medical director of Helena Women's Health in San Jose, California, and medical advisor to this book. A double temperature spike indicates that the hormonal sequence that leads to the successful release of an egg is out of order.

The symptothermal method (STM). Women who use this approach observe more than one fertility indicator, most commonly BBT and cervical mucus. One approach to STM is Weschler's Fertility Awareness Method (FAM), which has a woman monitor her BBT, mucus, and the position of her cervix. Log on to www.tcoyf.com for more on FAM.

Another method, the Natural Fertility Management program, monitors BBT, mucus, and the lunar cycle. It was developed by Francesca Naish, N.D., a naturopath at Jocelyn Centre for Natural Fertility Management and Holistic Medicine in Sydney, Australia, and author of *Healthy Parents, Healthy Babies* and *Natural Fertility*. (Dr. Naish believes there's a connection between a woman's fertility and the phases of the moon, a link that most other fertility experts discount.) Check out her Web site at www.fertility.com.au.

If you want a more complete picture of your fertility or are having trouble conceiving, STM is the way to go, says Weschler. No single clue can tell your entire reproductive story, she explains. And should you have as-yet-undiagnosed fertility problems, checking more than one fertility sign may help you pinpoint problems earlier.

"That's the beauty of this method. If you did have a fertility problem, you'd be eons ahead of everyone else," says Weschler. "If you don't get pregnant after three cycles of perfectly timed intercourse, you can bring in your chart and tell your doctor whether you're ovulating and the length of your luteal phase [the number of days after ovulation until menstruation starts]."

Luteal phases that are 12 days long or less are a sign that you should seek the advice of a fertility specialist, adds Dr. Metzger. Other signs that might indicate a problem include cycles that are consistently shorter than 26 days or that vary greatly in length from month to month.

If you suspect a problem, "the one thing you don't want to do is wait a year, especially if you're older," emphasizes Weschler.

If you decide to try STM, the Natural Family Planning Chart on page 186, which is provided by the Institute for Reproductive Health at Georgetown University School of Medicine in Washington, D.C., is a great way to track changes in BBT, cervical secretions, and the position of the cervix. The first copy of the chart has been filled in to illustrate how a typical cycle might look. To track your own cycle, make copies of the blank chart and follow these instructions.

Begin on the first day you get your period. First, subtract 19 from the number of days in the shortest of your last six cycles. Then draw a vertical line before this day on the chart. Next, take your temperature each morning upon awakening. Put a dot in the middle of the square that corresponds to your temperature for that day. Connect the dots each day with

(continued on page 188)

Natural Family Planning Chart

Month & Year _May/June 03_

Cycle Length

# of days in shortest of last 6 cycles   _28_

minus 19 =   _9_

Draw a vertical line before this day

Length of this cycle =   _31_

Temperature

Time of taking temperature   _7 am_

Basal Body Temperature (Fahrenheit)

99.0 / .9 / .8 / .7 / .6 / .5 / .4 / .3 / .2 / .1 / 98.0 / .9 / .8 / .7 / .6 / .5 / .4 / .3 / .2 / .1 / 97.0 / .9 / .8 / .7 / .6 / .5 / .4 / .3 / .2 / .1

Menstrual Cycle Day	Circle day of intercourse
Date	5/27 28 29 30 31 6/1 2 3 4 5 6 7 8 9 10 11 12 13 14 15 16 17 18 19 20 21 22 23 24 25 26 27

Menstrual Cycle Day: 1 2 3 4 5 6 7 8 9 10 11 12 13 14 15 16 17 18 19 20 21 22 23 24 25 26 27 28 29 30 31 32 33 34 35 36 37 38 39 40

Cervical Secretions (Feel, look, and touch)

Wet, slippery, transparent, or stretchy

Thick, cloudy, or sticky

Dry, no secretions seen or felt

Period

Cervix

High, soft, open

Low, firm, closed

Natural Family Planning Chart

Basal Body Temperature (Fahrenheit)

Month & Year _____

Cycle Length

\# of days in shortest of last 6 cycles _____

minus 19 = _____
Draw a vertical line before this day

Length of this cycle = _____

Temperature

Time of taking temperature _____

Menstrual Cycle Day	1	2	3	4	5	6	7	8	9	10	11	12	13	14	15	16	17	18	19	20	21	22	23	24	25	26	27	28	29	30	31	32	33	34	35	36	37	38	39	40
Circle day of intercourse																																								
Date																																								
Cervical Secretions (Feel, look, and touch) — Wet, slippery, transparent, or stretchy																																								
Thick, cloudy, or sticky																																								
Dry, no secretions seen or felt																																								
Period																																								
Cervix — High, soft, open																																								
Low, firm, closed																																								

Temperature scale (top to bottom): 99.0, .9, .8, .7, .6, .5, .4, .3, .2, .1, 98.0, .9, .8, .7, .6, .5, .4, .3, .2, .1, 97.0

a straight line. After the first 10 days of the cycle, draw a horizontal line on the rule just above the highest of the normal low temperatures recorded. This is the cover line. When your temperature goes above this line, draw a vertical line just before the temperature rise. For tracking purposes, your most fertile days are the days between the two vertical lines.

In addition to tracking changes in your basal body temperature, also

FERTILITY VISIONARIES

Francesca Naish, N.D., and Natural Fertility Management

When naturopath Francesca Naish was first mulling over her birth control options, it was the swinging sixties, the era defined by free love and the Pill. Ironically, the method that most appealed to her was the least fashionable: monitoring her natural signs of fertility. Figuring there must be kindred soul sisters out there, she opened a small practice in Sydney, Australia, to spread the word about natural contraception, like monitoring changes in cervical mucus and basal body temperature (BBT).

"But it soon became evident that there was also a need for *conception* information," she recalls. "And as my studies and practice grew, so did the increase in fertility problems." According to Dr. Naish, the women who came to her seemed starved for holistic approaches to *all* their reproductive needs.

Thirty years later, Dr. Naish's practice has evolved into an international company, Natural Fertility Management (NFM). It advocates using fertility awareness methods for natural birth control and conception and offers holistic preconception care and natural fertility treatments.

Dr. Naish continues to treat patients at her Jocelyn Centre in Sydney, but NFM also has more than 1,000 accredited practitioners in the United States, Canada, and elsewhere. Thousands of unaffiliated practitioners use Dr. Naish's methods in their practices, and her books, including *Natural Fertility* and *Healthy Parents, Better Babies*, have helped millions of couples boost fertility on their own.

"We typically see professional couples in their late thirties or early forties who have delayed having a child until later in life," says Dr. Naish. "Infertility is the major reason they come to us, though we're gratified to find an increasing number coming in for preconception health care *before* they try to conceive."

note the days on which you have intercourse and the consistency of your cervical secretions. As ovulation approaches and you enter your fertile period, your cervical secretions will become more abundant, slippery, and clearer. They may also stretch 2 or more inches between your thumb and forefinger.

If you choose to monitor the position of your cervix, note those days

During the initial visit, Dr. Naish (and doctors who use her approach) assesses a couple's reproductive and general health. Included in the assessment: tests for genitourinary infections, possible exposure to toxins, and nutritional deficiencies, all of which affect male and female fertility. Couples are advised on diet, exercise, and stress management and taught to chart fertility signs. "All those considering conception are given nutritional support, and herbal remedies are used to treat any reproductive health issues, whether or not the couple is experiencing fertility problems," says Dr. Naish. "Allergy, *Candida*, and digestive and immune system disorders are investigated and treated naturally. In some cases, other alternative therapies, such as acupuncture, homeopathy, osteopathy, and hypnotherapy, are also used. In vitro fertilization or other assisted reproductive technologies are seen as a last resort," she explains.

NFM's success rate is high, although exact numbers aren't available. (Research is currently under way.) But one study of a preconception program similar to NFM promoted by Foresight: The Association for the Promotion of Preconceptual Care, which is based in the United Kingdom, found that more than 80 percent of previously infertile couples got pregnant after 2 years.

Contact information: For names of accredited NFM practitioners and information on ordering Dr. Naish's Conscious Conception kit (which includes a copy of *Natural Fertility*, instructions on charting fertility signs, a relaxation tape, and guidelines for preconception care), visit her Web site at www.fertility.com.au or write to The Jocelyn Centre for Natural Fertility Management and Holistic Medicine, 1/46 Grosvenor Street, Woollahra Sydney NSW 2025, Australia. E-mail Dr. Naish at jocelyncentre@fertility.com.au.

when your cervix is soft, open, and higher as possible fertile days. In addition to filling out the chart, you might find it helpful to note in your personal calendar or planner any schedule changes or disturbances from your normal routine. Having a record of such changes—including days you woke up early, were traveling, or were under a lot of stress—can be helpful in explaining any irregularities in your chart.

Calendar or rhythm method. Devised in the 1930s, this approach works on the assumption that sperm and egg are viable for 6 days and ovulation occurs on day 14, plus or minus 2 days. It's quite simple: You just chart your cycle on a calendar to identify the days on which you're most likely to ovulate. To use this method, you first have to determine your baseline cycle length—which means that you must record the length of at least six menstrual cycles to find your shortest and longest cycles. (A cycle begins on day 1 of your period and lasts until the day before your next period.)

Once you've identified the length of these six cycles, subtract 19 (days) from the shortest cycle. That's your first fertile day. (For example, if your shortest cycle was 26 days, your first fertile day would be day 7.) To figure your last fertile day, subtract 11 days from your longest cycle (day 19 of a 30-day cycle, for instance). Thus, if your period starts on October 3, consider yourself fertile from October 9 to October 21.

While many women swear by this method, most fertility experts don't recommend it, particularly if you're having trouble conceiving. "It's guesswork," explains Dr. Stanford.

A variation on the calendar approach, the Standard Days Method, can be used by women whose cycles are from 26 to 32 days long—that's about 80 percent of all women. In this method, you track your fertile days using a ring of 32 beads called CycleBeads. Each CycleBead represents one day of your cycle. The beads are color-coded to indicate whether you're on a fertile or infertile day.

Each day, you move a tiny rubber ring to a new bead. When your period starts (day 1), you put the rubber ring on the red bead. The next six beads are brown, indicating you're infertile. Beads 8 through 19 are white, meaning you're probably fertile. On day 20, beads become brown again until your next period, when you start over with the red bead. For more information on CycleBeads, log on to www.cyclebeads.com.

Ovulation prediction and detection kits. Most kits available in drugstores haven't been studied long enough to accurately assess their effectiveness. But if monitoring mucus and daily temperature readings isn't your thing, this high-tech approach is an option, says Dr. Stanford. Most of these kits measure LH in your urine, which usually surges the day before or day of ovulation. Remember, though, that if you wait until you're ovulating when you have intercourse, your partner's sperm may miss your egg. According to Dr. Stanford's research, the Clear Plan Easy Fertility Monitor measures both LH and estrogen and provides good advance warning that ovulation is approaching, making it perhaps the most accurate kit now available. The downside: Clear Plan costs about $200, plus the cost of urine test sticks.

13

Conception-Specific Sex

Here's the ultimate conception scenario: Soft music fills the room as you and your partner enjoy a candlelight dinner. You laugh, dance, and finally tumble into bed for a night of high-octane lovemaking that puts even the Kama Sutra to shame. A few weeks later, still aglow from that heated night, you get the best news of all. You're pregnant.

In a perfect world, all babies would be conceived this way. In the real world, though, those wild nights of supersonic, multiposition sex could be dimming your conception odds.

GET BACK TO BASICS

"We laugh in the office about couples swinging from chandeliers or shaking a dead chicken around the bed three times," says Scott J. Roseff, M.D., director of the West Essex Center for Advanced Reproductive Endocrinology in West Orange, New Jersey, and clinical associate professor in the obstetrics and gynecology department at the University of Medicine and Dentistry of New Jersey. There's little science behind the best sexual techniques for conceiving, "but if you want semen to get where it needs to go, there are certain things that make sense," he notes.

That's not to say that you and your partner won't get pregnant after a hot night of sexual acrobatics or that you can't continue to experiment in bed. You might want to tone it down for a while, however, particularly if you're having trouble getting pregnant. Go ahead and indulge in romantic dinners and music, but consider forgoing the chandeliers—as well as a few other conception-busting sexual habits. Here are some baby-making basics that just might make a difference.

Focus on foreplay. Put away those commercial lubricants, like K-Y Jelly, which can diminish sperm function and may even kill the little swimmers outright. Instead, concentrate on your lead-in to sex. Lots of cuddling and stimulation beforehand should give you all the vaginal lubrication you need for satisfying sex, plus provide sperm some added juice for their swim to the finish.

If after foreplay you still need a lubrication jump start, water—particularly purified bottled water—may be your safest bet. Some experts recommend saliva, but because it contains bacteria, it can injure or kill sperm. "The human mouth is the most bacteria-laden organ of the body," notes Dr. Roseff.

Enjoy a nightcap—of cough syrup. Cough syrups that contain the active ingredient guaifenesin, such as Robitussin, soften and thin nasal mucus to clear clogged respiratory passages. Theoretically, guaifenesin also thins cervical mucus, helping sperm to glide and thrive in your reproductive system. No studies have been done, but some couples report success.

Experts agree that taking a dose of cough syrup several hours before intercourse is relatively harmless and may help. Because your cervical mucus should thin and soften on its own around the time of ovulation, however, such outside aid may be unnecessary. (See chapter 12 for more information on mucus patterns throughout your cycle.)

Caution: If you decide to kick off your night with cough syrup, make sure it's not an antihistamine, which may have the opposite of the desired effect, leaving your mucous membranes high and dry.

Go on a mission. Some sexual positions may be highly arousing, but they're duds when it comes to keeping sperm in your reproductive tract and within reach of a fertilizable egg. Your best bet is probably an old standard, the missionary position (woman lying on her back, man on top). "The way the female reproductive tract is designed, things tend to run down the vagina and into the cervix when a woman is on her back," notes Dr. Roseff. "When she's sitting on top (with the man lying on his back) or standing, gravity takes over and sperm runs out."

For deeper penetration, place a pillow in the small of your back under your hips to boost them up, so your partner's penis reaches closer to your cervix and there's a downward flow of sperm. Another good position: Have your partner enter you from behind while you're kneeling on your hands and knees, also called doggie style. Don't stand or sit up right away, though, because sperm may escape.

Discover the big "G." Having an orgasm is certainly key to your sexual pleasure, but not necessarily key to conception (your partner's orgasms are more important conception-wise, since without ejaculation, there's no sperm—and no baby). That said, your orgasm probably still matters, particularly the kind you have. Sex researcher Beverly Whipple, R.N., Ph.D., professor emerita of nursing at Rutgers University and coauthor of the bestseller *The G Spot and Other Recent Discoveries about Human Sexuality*, believes that orgasms via G-spot stimulation are more likely to result in conception than orgasms via clitoral stimulation (although no formal studies have been done). "We've observed that when there's G-spot stimulation, the uterus pushes down into the vagina and the cervix dips into the seminal pool," Dr. Whipple notes. "During clitoral stimulation, the uterus pulls up."

The G-spot, or Grafenberg spot, is a highly sensitive area of tissue and nerve endings on the upper wall of the vagina a few inches back from the vaginal opening toward the cervix. The clitoris is located under the soft inner lips, called the labia minora, that surround the vagina and the opening of your urethra. To find the G-spot, have your partner insert one or two fingers into your vagina with his palm facing up until he finds a raised spot or ridges that feel rougher than surrounding tissue. He should then stroke the spot using a beckoning gesture or try stimulating it with his penis during intercourse. Most women find this highly pleasurable, although some report an urge to urinate.

Try selective ejaculation. The idea that ejaculating too often lowers sperm counts has been debated for years. Some say frequent ejaculations diminish only the volume of ejaculate, not the number of sperm. Others, though, believe that sperm totals shrink, too.

Bottom line: Go ahead and have sex as much as you like throughout your cycle, but if your partner has a low sperm count or you just want to boost your baby-making chances, try slowing it down to every other day or every 3 days during your 5- to 6-day fertile window. This may help build your partner's sperm reserves.

Take a break from oral and anal sex. Variety may be the spice of life, but when it comes to baby-making, oral and anal sex are probably best saved for after conception. They can introduce harmful bacteria into your vagina via saliva or feces, causing fertility-robbing infections that keep you from full reproductive health and prevent your partner's sperm from reaching your eggs. (See chapter 10 for more on the fertility risks of infections and illness.)

Stay sperm-friendly. "Your vagina is healthiest when it's clean, dry, and exposed to air," says Dr. Roseff. "When it's dark and restricted, the acid–alkaline balance is thrown off."

Good strategies for keeping your vagina healthy and his sperm happy include:

* Avoiding tight clothing, including panty hose.

* Wearing cotton underwear instead of nylon

* Wiping your genital area from front to back instead of vice versa.

* Limiting your consumption of fat, sugar, and carbohydrates, and eating plenty of yogurt that contains active acidophilus cultures.

* Boosting your immune system with adequate sleep, exercise, and antioxidant vitamins, including vitamins C and E.

Give up douching. No matter how you look at it, douching is the "biggest no-no on the planet for women," says Dr. Roseff. Douching before sex can throw off your vagina's acid–alkaline balance, which for sperm is akin to landing on an inhospitable planet without life support. And douching immediately after sex may flush out sperm and even kill them. What's more, douching sometimes forces bacteria up into your reproductive tract, increasing your chances of infection, including fertility-robbing pelvic inflammatory disease, or PID.

DON'T FORGET THE FUN

If you've read chapter 12, you've learned to pinpoint your fertile days. And you just read what works in the bedroom and what doesn't. So you're ready to make a baby, right?

Not necessarily. For some couples, making love on schedule with a list of sexual do's and don'ts has about as much spontaneity and passion as a military drill. And if you have been trying unsuccessfully for a while or are undergoing fertility treatment, sex can become even more of a perfunctory means to an end rather than the loving centerpiece of your relationship.

"Sex and conception were not meant to be mechanical utilitarian acts, but healthy, fertile, life-affirming connections between loving partners," notes certified professional midwife Aviva Romm, president of the American Herbalists Guild and author of several books, including *Natural Health and Birth*.

"Keep it fun," adds family physician Richard Roberts, M.D., J.D., professor of family medicine at the University of Wisconsin Medical School in Madison. "Keep a sense of spontaneity. If it feels like work, you've killed something precious."

Indeed, the time in your life when you're planning a family is the time to really connect with your partner and strengthen your bond. Even if you never conceive, it will deepen your love and sustain your relationship. And if you eventually do get pregnant, having a solid relationship will certainly add to your baby's sense of security and well-being and may even boost your parenting skills.

"You have 18 years to raise this child," Dr. Roberts notes. "If you stay committed to developing a communication style that lets you keep things out in the open, those are skill sets that will serve you well in the years ahead."

PRACTICAL GOALS, SCINTILLATING SEX

When Duke University Medical Center psychologist Jennifer E. Norten, Ph.D., recently asked 88 women and 27 men who were being treated for infertility about their sex lives, she was surprised by the disconnect between their perceptions of their sex lives and sexual reality. A significant proportion of the women (the sample size of men was too small to be statistically significant) reported having less intercourse, less sexual desire, and generally less satisfying sexual relationships with their partners. Yet the numbers suggested that most were actually making love about as frequently as couples who weren't undergoing infertility treatment.

"Even though they were still having sex as often, they weren't enjoying it as much," notes Dr. Norten, clinical professor in the medical center's reproductive medicine program in Durham, North Carolina. "Part of the issue is their perception," she says. Couples get so focused on sex for procreation that making love becomes a source of tension rather than joy.

Here are a few simple strategies to add some pizzazz to your baby-making efforts and keep you from falling into the sexual and relationship doldrums.

Take time for intimacy, not just sex. "A lot of women who are going through infertility feel like a failure, and sex triggers those feelings," notes Dr. Norten. In order to enjoy their sex lives, "women really need to feel good about themselves and feel close to their partners," she says.

One way is to carve out nonsexual time for you and your partner to share activities you both enjoy or just to be romantic. "You have to look at intimacy as more than intercourse," Dr. Norten advises. "Go out to dinner. Have foreplay that doesn't always lead to sex."

Relaxing together without stressful sexual expectations may even lead to super sex later on. "The greatest aphrodisiac is in the mind," says Susan Taylor, Ph.D., a nutritional biochemist in Newburyport, Massachusetts, and author of *Sexual Radiance*. "Make a date and take time during the week to prepare your minds. Say, 'Saturday we'll spend the day together—not necessarily to have sex—and see what happens.'"

Strive for spiritual connection. Emotional intimacy often lays the groundwork for a deeper spiritual bond between you and your partner, which, in turn, strengthens your sexual relationship. Do things that inspire you both to higher levels of awareness, such as meditating together, attending religious services, or even sharing a walk in the forest.

If you're looking for a unique way to strengthen your spiritual connection with your partner, the two of you might want to take a class so you can practice tantric yoga techniques together, suggests yoga and physical therapist Nataly Pluta, P.T., A.Y.T., a physical therapist and yoga therapist who runs Pluta Movement Therapeutics in Del Mar, California. Couples stand looking at one another while holding yoga poses and breathing in synch. The aim is to open the flow of healing energy to both partners' lower chakras, centered around their reproductive organs (according to Eastern healing traditions, the body has seven chakras, or spiritual energy centers, each corresponding to a different region of the body).

"It's not sexual," notes Pluta. "We get them breathing on the same wavelength, so that they'll be on the same spiritual wavelength as they're going through infertility and, hopefully, pregnancy together."

Communicate, communicate, communicate. "When there are problems in the bedroom, you really need to keep the lines of communication open," says Linda D. Applegarth, Ed.D., director of psychological services at the Center for Reproductive Medicine and Infertility and clinical assistant professor of psychology at New York Presbyterian Hospital–Weill Medical College of Cornell University in New York City. Because of the intimate nature of such problems, it's especially important to approach them from the standpoint of mutual respect and support for each other.

For example, before starting a potentially emotional discussion, consider the timing. Pick times when you're both relaxed and clearheaded. "Don't confront him the minute he comes in the door or call from work to say, 'Our sex life is a mess,'" Dr. Applegarth advises. "Good communication requires gentleness and delicacy. Show that what you're saying comes out of caring about the relationship." If you find that talking with each other is becoming increasingly difficult, don't be afraid to get third-party professional help, urges Dr. Applegarth.

Get a life. Sometimes you're so focused on the fact that you're not getting pregnant, you spend all your time talking and obsessing about it with your partner. Learning to compartmentalize those feelings can ease the strain and lighten your relationship. "Schedule a couple's meeting—a specific time to talk about it," suggests Dr. Norten. "The rest of the time, lead your life as usual."

Let go of fear. Though it has never been proven, mind–body medicine suggests that worrying about problems, including infertility, may act like a self-fulfilling prophecy. In other words, the body may manifest the mind's deepest fears. The key is to relax and stop trying to control things.

Dr. Taylor recalls directing one infertile patient to close her eyes and imagine going into her womb: "I asked her what she saw and she said, 'I see darkness—I'm scared I'm not going to get pregnant.'" Notes Dr. Taylor, "You're never going to accept sperm if you see darkness." Chapters 6, 7, and 18 offer tips on dealing with stress and destructive emotions that may compromise your fertility.

Don't forget your nonfertile times. Scheduling lovemaking dates when you're not fertile or just jumping into bed spontaneously is as important to your relationship as timing is to baby-making. "Make it known when intercourse isn't for procreation, so there will still be an association of sex as fun and recreation," Dr. Applegarth advises.

Feel free to fantasize. Sharing sexual fantasies is another way to spruce up sagging libidos. The key is being totally honest about your fantasies and open to hearing your partner's, even the most erotic ones. Don't worry if you're squeamish about acting them out; talking about them can be almost as good.

HERBAL APHRODISIACS AND OTHER SEXUAL STIMULANTS

Herbal stimulants are a good way to fire up your libido, but remember that your goal is a healthy baby. For this reason, avoid "under-the-counter" stimulants, such as Spanish fly, a powder derived from insects, which contains a potentially deadly ingredient called cantharidin. Yohimbe, a popular herbal sexual stimulant for men, is known to cause hallucinations, dizziness, and rapid heartbeat in high doses and therefore should probably be avoided, too.

Try gentler aphrodisiacs for baby-making, recommends certified professional midwife Aviva Romm, president of the American Herbalists Guild and author of several books, including *Natural Health and Birth*. Even something as simple as eating spicy foods can heighten your senses—and your sexual desire. For example, consider adding ginger to a romantic candlelit meal. Ginger gently boosts circulation, including circulation to your genitals, and creates a warm blood-rush sensation throughout the body for up to 2 hours.

Like spicy foods, scary movies and thrillers also heighten the senses. So do aromatherapy candles and oils. Romm suggests either surprising your partner with a new fragrance or taking him along with you on your next shopping trip so he can help pick out a scent you both find stimulating. Fragrances said to kindle both male and female libidos include jasmine, vanilla, ylang-ylang, sandalwood, and patchouli.

Place aromatherapy candles near your bed, bath, or favorite lovemaking spot to get you both in the mood. Or try adding aromatherapy essential oils to a candlelit bath or using them as a massage oil. To get you started, here's a recipe for a libido-lifting massage oil recommended by Romm.

Sensuality Oil

This aromatherapy oil can be used both in your bath and as a massage oil. The sandalwood and vanilla essential oils can be costly but are a worthwhile treat. Store the mixture away from direct heat and light.

- 3½   ounces pure almond oil
- ¼   ounce sandalwood essential oil
- ¼   ounce vanilla essential oil

Mix the almond oil with the sandalwood and vanilla essential oils. Add 1 teaspoon to your bathwater or use as needed for massage.

"Sharing fantasies taps into the erotic aspects of the brain," says Marvin A. Stone, M.D., adjunct professor of psychiatry at the University of Texas Health Sciences Center at Houston and author of *Close Encounters: 100 Tips for Intimacy*. "It stimulates pleasurable brain chemicals like dopamine and makes you the most powerful erotic stimulant in your partner's life. Your partner will want to keep coming back because he knows you're the source of opening him up to his fantasy world."

Savor a sensual massage. This is different from a regular shoulder or back massage. The aim is for you and your partner to touch each other lightly, using a feather, the tips of your fingers, or anything that grabs your fancy, to arouse one another but not to orgasm. Touch your partner's entire body, concentrating on sexually sensitive areas, including the inner thighs and genitals.

"At the same time, you can engage in erotic talk and fantasies," Dr. Stone suggests. "When you draw things out over hours this way, your orgasm is much more powerful."

Get out of the bedroom. If you've always fantasized about making love to the sound of ocean waves or in the back of a pickup truck under the stars, this is the time to indulge yourself.

"Often it feels like your doctors are in the bedroom, waiting to do a postcoital test," Dr. Applegarth explains. "It's hard to get those people out of your psyche." Trying someplace new is a good way to leave behind fertility frustrations that may be associated with your regular lovemaking environment and put the spice back into sexual encounters that have gone stale from overscheduling and stress.

14

A Fertility-Revving Lifestyle

Leslie Keefe thought that she embraced the kind of lifestyle that would foster a pregnancy. She didn't smoke or drink. She walked regularly with friends, had a strong relationship with her husband, and cooked low-fat, balanced meals based on plenty of fruits and vegetables. After 8 years of trying to conceive, Leslie and her husband began to assume that the cancer treatment she had endured years earlier may have rendered her infertile. Since they weren't interested in high-tech infertility treatment, they were coming to accept the fate of a child-free life. Yet one month after the couple spent 3 weeks on an extended family reunion at the New Jersey shore, Leslie learned she would have her first child at the age of 38!

Although Leslie's lifestyle was basically healthy, she believes her fertility wasn't actually *revved up* until a number of small factors came together. She got a little more sleep than usual, spent more time around loved ones, and was surrounded by the elements that boosted her mood and energy.

"Just looking at a picture of the ocean has a positive effect on me, and here I was in the water every day," she explains. "It makes sense that between reliving my happy childhood memories at the beach and the intense sunshine, I was finally able to conceive," says the graphics designer from Bethlehem, Pennsylvania.

If you're already following the preconception plan that's outlined in the preceding chapters, you and your partner are taking pretty good care of yourselves by now. You may have already made major improvements in your diet, environment, and emotional and physical health. Now, as you're actively trying to conceive, more subtle refinements enter the plan.

Lifestyle factors concerning your work schedules and the temperature of your baths may seem like minor issues. But in this chapter, you'll learn why these and other nuances in your habits and surroundings can influence how easily you conceive. Think of it this way: The sperm and egg maturing in your bodies right now may be the very ones that will form your future child. Because of this, it's important to lead a lifestyle that's healthy and balanced all the way down to the cellular level. Read on to learn how.

MAKE THE MOST OF SLEEP AND SUNLIGHT

According to the National Sleep Foundation, 70 percent of Americans don't get enough sleep, and most sleep disorder sufferers remain undiagnosed and untreated. Yet sleep is integral to our quality of life, overall health, and fertility.

Sleep helps restore and rejuvenate the brain and organ systems—including the reproductive system. When sleep suffers over the long run, so does our relationship with our spouse, our mood, our immunity, and even our hormone balance. Sleep loss can also lead to fertility-disrupting lifestyle factors like caffeine overuse and weight gain.

Lack of sleep may even lead to menstrual irregularity—a factor that can delay the time it takes to conceive. When researchers polled women in notoriously sleep-deprived professions—flight attendants and nurses working the late shift—*half* of the women reported irregular menstrual cycles (compared to about 20 percent of the general population). Some stopped ovulating altogether.

Even the light we are exposed to on a day-to-day basis has an influence on ovulation and reproductive hormones—one that has fascinated (and perplexed) researchers for years. "There is some evidence that before the age of artificial lighting, birth control pills, and working indoors, women all ovulated in sync with the phases of the moon," says Joyce Stahmann, M.P.H., a fertility educator and professional herbalist in Portland, Oregon, who teaches the Natural Fertility Management Program.

Similarly, researchers at the University of California, San Diego, Sleep Lab have successfully been able to alter the length of women's menstrual cycles by exposing women to artificial light around the middle of their cycles, while they slept. It appears that the hormones that trigger ovulation, and even the sperm maturation process, are somehow tied into the body's biological clock, explains Daniel Kripke, M.D., the current director of the Sleep Lab, who oversaw some of this research. Dr. Kripke is a world-famous circadian rhythm expert and a professor of psychiatry at the university.

The calibrated release of sleep–wake hormones such as melatonin and cortisol is triggered, in part, by information given to the brain by its "light meter," the pineal gland. Since the same part of the brain that regulates sleep–wake hormones also stimulates daily pulses of reproductive hormones for men and women, scientists suspect some feedback between these systems. Another concern is the effect that natural light can have on mood. "Lack of sunlight can result in depression, which in turn can suppress fertility," notes Dr. Kripke.

Because sleep and daylight are integral to our biological clocks, it's important to get sufficient amounts of both. Here are some guidelines.

Honor your personal sleep needs. Although the optimal amount of sleep is about 8 hours on average, requirements vary from person to person and somewhat from season to season. "You are probably skimping on the amount of sleep you need if you have signs of drowsiness or poor concentration during the day," says Stahmann.

Get outdoors. Shoot for an hour or more out in sunlight each day, even if you have to split it up with a 10-minute walk in the morning, lunch on the patio, and a quick Frisbee toss with your dog in the late afternoon. If

WHAT WORKED FOR US
SHE CHANGED HER WORKLOAD AND LEARNED HOW TO "NEST"

Jan McLeod spent more than 8 years building client rapport and staff respect as a sales manager. Her career seemed to be going so well that she didn't want to change anything. But after 3½ years of trying to get pregnant, she and her husband had to be honest. When fertility evaluations confirmed that nothing was physically wrong, she took a closer look at her lifestyle.

"My father-in-law spoke up and said that if my focus was totally on my career and not on my home life, it could hold me back from getting pregnant because my body could sense that I wasn't ready. At first I resented his remarks, but eventually I came to believe he was right," Jan recalls.

"When I thought about it, I was constantly trying to change my workload or strategize better because I was so fatigued," she says. Jan didn't want to lose her company benefits, but she knew she was burned out from the pressure of making demanding budgets month after month. When a lower-profile job opened up in another department, she jumped on it.

Jan had to give up the glamour of travel and the creative charge she got when brainstorming her sales pitches. But with a more manageable workload, she found a different kind of satisfaction. "I was now working with a lot of nurturing women, rather than the more competitive group in my old department," she notes. And she could spend more time being involved with her church and family. Within 2 months at her new job, Jan conceived. After having her daughter, she continued to work part-time. Seven months later, she became pregnant with a son.

"I discovered that taking a step back at work can be a step forward for fertility. It's not that you have to slam the breaks on your career, but a priority shift made all the difference for me," says the mother of two.

time or weather constraints force you to stay indoors, Dr. Kripke recommends the use of a light box, a portable unit that allows you to get light even while indoors and is often used for the treatment of seasonal affective disorder (SAD). You can purchase a light box through any of the numerous online stores that offer them for sale. (For more information on light boxes, you can log on to Dr. Kripke's Web site, www.brightenyourlife.info.)

Don't work odd hours if you can help it. "A growing body of evidence suggests that late night and overnight work schedules are associated with menstrual irregularities, reproductive disturbances, and risk of adverse pregnancy," says Phyllis Zee, M.D., Ph.D., director of the Sleep Disorders Center and associate professor of neurology at Northwestern University Medical School in Chicago. Ideally, men and women should opt out of shiftwork while they're trying to conceive, and women should also try to avoid it while they're pregnant. If you must do shiftwork, be vigilant about getting sufficient rest and recuperation in your hours away from the job, Dr. Zee advises.

Keep your sleep and wake time consistent. Try to go to bed and get up at the same time every day, even on weekends. The luxury of "sleeping in" comes at a high price, warns Dr. Kripke. It may actually make you groggier, plus it's harder to go to bed on Sunday night and get up on Monday.

Still your mind. Before bed, avoid paying bills, reading books or watching movies with troubling story lines, and any other activities that could keep your mind racing rather than relaxing into a peaceful sleep. Instead, make a habit out of nightly calming rituals like spiritual reflection and partner massage.

Adjust your lighting. Turning down dimmer switches and using low-wattage bulbs in the evening are helpful for someone who has trouble falling asleep. On the other hand, if you develop sleep deficiency because you awaken too early, brighter light in the evening may shift your body clock so that you stay asleep longer, says Dr. Kripke.

Keep a space cushion between stimulants and sleep. Both caffeine and alcohol are discouraged when you're trying to get pregnant, but if you do occasionally indulge, limit your use to more than 5 hours before bedtime. "Even though it may feel as though alcohol helps you fall asleep, it actually disturbs your sleep," notes circadian rhythm researcher Elizabeth Klerman, M.D., assistant professor of medicine at Brigham and Women's Hospital in Boston.

Stay away from melatonin supplements. "Although it's tempting to self-treat insomnia or jet lag with melatonin supplements, it's not a good idea for any man or woman who is trying to conceive," says Dr. Kripke. "There is a risk of suppressed fertility and even gonadal atrophy in people who take melatonin supplements."

Be honest about sleep disorders. The National Sleep Foundation offers symptom lists and self-evaluations to help you identify sleep disorders such as insomnia, sleep apnea, and restless legs syndrome. Log on to the Web site www.sleepfoundation.org for more information. If you suspect that you have a sleep disorder, see your doctor—but make sure she knows that you're trying to conceive so you don't receive contraindicating medications.

PLAY IT COOL

"The testicles hang outside of a man's body for a reason. Sperm are optimally produced and maintained at a temperature that's lower than the body core," explains reproductive endocrinologist and gynecologic surgeon Deborah Metzger, M.D., Ph.D., medical director of Helena Women's Health in San Jose, California, and medical advisor to this book.

The skin sac holding the sperm-producing testicles, known as the scrotum, acts as a kind of temperature-control system by loosening up when body temperature increases so that the testicles can hang slightly farther from the body. Similarly, the scrotum constricts to bring the testicles closer to a man's warm abdomen when it's really cold outside.

Sperm's sensitivity to high temperatures is why higher rates of delayed conception are reported in men with occupations that involve welding (where the temperature in the room is high) or driving (where prolonged sitting prevents airflow to the testicles). "Just an increase of 2 to 4 degrees Fahrenheit in the testes can result in numerous sperm abnormalities, including the inability to swim properly and low count," explains Philip Werthman, M.D., a urologist specializing in male infertility and microsurgery who is the director of the Center for Male Reproductive Medicine and chief of urology at Center City Hospital, both in Los Angeles. Men with cryptorchidism or varicoceles must be particularly committed to heat-related lifestyle modifications, since these conditions already impair thermoregulation. (See chapters 2 and 17 for more information on these abnormalities.)

Men who habitually take long baths, nightly soaks in a hot tub, or leisurely breaks in steam rooms are encouraged to quit at least 2½ months before they want to conceive. (It takes that long for a man to produce a new "crop" of sperm that haven't been damaged by the heat.) It's also important to stop using electric blankets and heating a waterbed—unless you just warm the bed and turn off the heating unit before you get in.

Male fertility can be impaired by less extreme circumstances than oven-like environments, however. Anything that holds the testicles close to the body and restricts airflow to the genitals challenges the sperm's temperature-regulating system. Looser pants are better than restrictive clothing such as tight jeans and leather pants while you're trying to reproduce, notes Dr. Werthman. And while athletic supporters and bicycle shorts keep the genitals safe, it's recommended that you take them off promptly after exercising to prevent any additional heating they might cause.

When it comes to underwear, boxers theoretically offer better cooling capacity and airflow than briefs. But since few studies can document any undershort-related change in spermatogenesis, most experts leave it to personal choice. Fertility experts do, however, advise men to think about the *material* that covers their gonads. Nylon, polyester, and other artificial fibers cause gonadal temperatures to rise more easily than cotton. Researchers in one study found that a tight, polyester covering over the testes caused such consistent azoospermia (absence of sperm production) that they proposed this polyester "sling" as a new form of male contraception. Need another reason to stick with cotton? Materials that allow the genitals to breathe and stay cool offer protection against infections (like jock itch and candidiasis) for both men and women, says Dr. Werthman.

Does a woman also need to worry about overheating when she's trying to conceive? "Actually, yes," says Dr. Metzger. "The same mechanism that triggers miscarriage when a woman is sick with a fever could be triggered by other forms of excessive heat. Raising the internal body temperature with something like a hot tub, electric blanket, or running a marathon is going to be counterproductive around day 21 of her cycle when she's hoping for implantation," Dr. Metzger explains.

REDUCE RADIATION

Although the concept of "radiation" can be disconcerting, the human body itself produces a faint electromagnetic field (EMF) from the activity of nerves and organ systems. Low fields also occur naturally in the Earth's core and ripple through the sky during a lightning storm.

"There's some evidence that human beings may even need low-level EMF exposures in order to reproduce. They appear to play a role in the formation of new cells and organs, including spermatogenesis and fetal development," observes Henry Lai, Ph.D., research professor in the bioengineering department of the University of Washington in Seattle.

Electromagnetic radiation gets its charge from electric waves and magnetic waves moving together. Unfortunately, the fastest and strongest of these waves are destructive to living organisms because of their ionizing properties. For instance, nuclear weapons, nuclear power, and x-rays create charged particles called ions that are capable of breaking molecular bonds and shattering atoms. This effect on living tissue can damage cell structure, including DNA. Since ionizing radiation is "drawn" to the weakest-bonded cells—those with the highest rate of growth and division—a maturing sperm or ova and the tissue of a developing fetus are particularly vulnerable.

In response, some of the world's most well-established preconception care programs, such as Foresight and Natural Fertility Management, encourage men and women to avoid even low-level ionizing radiation in the 4 months preceding conception and encourage women to continue to do so during pregnancy. That means limiting x-rays and even airplane travel to only what is absolutely necessary. "Not only does flying expose people to naturally occurring cosmic radiation, but up in the thin atmosphere, the rays aren't buffered by anything that might prevent them from penetrating the human body," explains Stahmann.

The effects of non-ionizing EMFs such as radio frequencies, microwaves, lasers, and AC power on human biology aren't as clear. But many preconception experts have enough concerns to encourage reduced overall EMF exposure as part of a fertility-revving lifestyle. These experts point to studies like one in which researchers placed colonies of mice near a cluster of TV and radio broadcasting transmitters (so many that the area became known as "Antenna Park"). Gradually, the mice produced fewer offspring, so that by the fifth and sixth breeding cycles, nearly all of the mice within range of the radio frequency currents were infertile. On the other hand, the same colony of mice that bred out of range of the transmitters produced full litters for all six breeding cycles.

The 60-hertz frequencies that run most household appliances have been linked to tumor growth, hormone alterations, and biorhythm changes in laboratory experiments. Since little is known about everyday exposure to low EMFs, federal agencies coordinated efforts to produce the 5-year Electric and Magnetic Fields Research and Public Information Dissemination Program (1993–1997). Some links were found between EMFs and infertility, miscarriages, cancer, Alzheimer's disease, learning disabilities, and chronic fatigue syndrome. The federal agencies, however, didn't consider the evidence to be convincing or consistent enough to declare specific exposure limits. "On the other hand, the electromagnetic fields could not be confirmed as harmless," points out Dr. Lai.

Although it's impossible to "get off the grid" in this communications-dense, electric-powered world, experts offer simple steps to reduce overall exposure in your immediate environment.

Pull the plug occasionally. The AC power you get from a wall outlet uses currents that flow back and forth (alternate) between the power source and the appliance, creating a field that can weakly penetrate your body. Since DC power from batteries flows only one way, there's less conduction. One option is to use more battery-powered tools, electric razors, laptop computers, and so forth. And don't forget about the countless human-powered alternatives to everyday devices, including hand mixers, can openers, clotheslines, and typewriters, as well as solar-powered items like calculators and water pumps. Thousands of novel tools for the kitchen and workshop can be purchased through Lehman's Non-Electric Catalog. (See page 324 for ordering information.)

Distance yourself from appliances. How much radiation you get while using an appliance depends on the intensity as well as the duration of the exposure. As a general rule, standing back 3 to 4 feet can help because the intensity drops off with distance, says Dr. Lai. Of course, you have to stay close to electric knives and power tools, but it's worthwhile to step back from appliances like blenders and garbage disposals and to hold appliances like hair dryers and vacuum cleaners as far away from your body as possible.

Power down your sleeping zone. It's especially important to distance yourself from EMFs in the bedroom, where you spend close to half your time, says Howard Buttram, M.D., a board-certified expert in environmental medicine and internal medicine who practices the Foresight Program for Preconception Care at The Woodlands Healing Research Center in Quakertown, Pennsylvania. Rather than positioning clocks, radios, lamps, and baby monitors at your bedside, keep them on the other side of the room. Try to set up your bed away from electric outlets, too. Since air conditioners, fans, and portable electric heaters generate high EMFs, the best policy is to run them *before* you settle down in a room, then turn them off when you're going to bed, Dr. Buttram adds.

Limit office exposures. A study of 500 employees in the Midwest concluded that women who worked with computer monitors, or video display units (VDUs), were three and a half times more likely to have impaired fertility from endometriosis and two and a half times more likely to have cervical factor infertility (a condition in which the sperm has difficulty penetrating) than women who didn't work with monitors.

If your work involves using a computer, sit at least arm's length (30 inches) away from your monitor, and move away from it when you're involved with other tasks. You may also want to stick with newer, flat-panel monitors or laptop computer screens, which don't produce the rapid sawtooth waves that make VDUs a bigger concern, explains Dr. Lai. It's also wise to sit as far as possible from laser printers, copy machines, and modems, adds Dr. Buttram.

Test your home's radiation. If you're concerned about the EMFs running through your living area, you can purchase a gaussmeter or hire an environmental engineer to evaluate them, says Dr. Lai. "There's no clear cutoff point, but levels of 0.4 milligauss and under offer the best protection against nerve stimulation and possible cell penetration, in my opinion," he says. "If your home measures as high as 4 milligauss, you have reason for concern. Old wiring like the knob-and-tube style, or a nearby power line, could be to blame."

Keep away from high-voltage lines. Electricity on power lines can run between 50 and 765 kilovolts (kVs) until it reaches the transformer box near your home, which converts it into low-frequency AC power. It takes a distance of 200 feet for the magnetic fields of a 115-kV power line to drop to the "safer" 0.4 milligauss range recommended by Dr. Lai—and much larger distances for fields to drop off on higher-powered lines. "In general, don't live, work, or walk in close proximity to high-voltage lines," stresses Dr. Buttram. "Ideally, the areas of the home where you spend the most time should be the farthest distance from your transformer box and incoming telephone wires."

Take herbal protection against radiation. "Herbs can be extremely effective at reducing the effects of radiation on the body," says Stahmann. "My first recommendation for helping with radiation exposure is a good reishi mushroom extract (*Ganoderma lucidum*). Look for a product that contains a minimum of 10 percent polysaccharides and 4 percent triterpenes, and take between 800 and 2,400 milligrams a day," she says. Stay at the higher end of the dose if you're experiencing unexplained infertility, which could be due to the effects of radiation. You'll also want to take a larger dose if you know you have high exposures from frequent x-rays or you have an "electrical occupation," such as working in a power plant or working with radar, power tools, electronics, or television or broadcast equipment. Stahmann recommends taking the extract for 6 weeks on, then 1 week off, for as long as the high exposure is present.

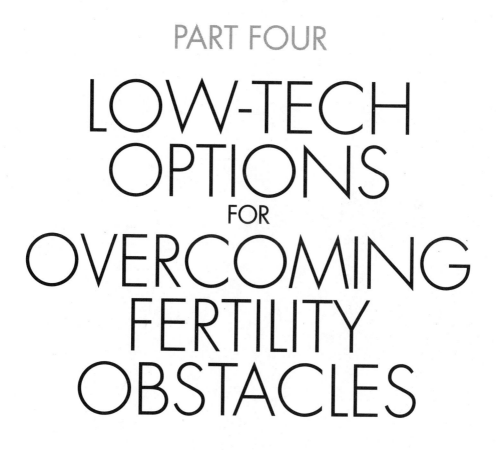

PART FOUR

LOW-TECH OPTIONS
FOR
OVERCOMING FERTILITY OBSTACLES

15

Getting to the Bottom of Fertility Problems

We spend most of our reproductive lives trying to keep our primordial life-giving capacity on a leash. So it's only natural to expect all that procreative power we've been holding back with pills, condoms, and diaphragms to gush out and work its magic soon after we set aside birth control. And for the great majority of couples, it does. Eighty-five percent of couples can discontinue contraception, have intercourse during the time that ovulation prediction methods indicate, and conceive before a year is up.

Even couples considered "subfertile" may very well have the capability to conceive but just don't do so in the first year of trying. Half of them conceive in the second year instead. Providence, your biology, your environment—all may play roles. So when conception is delayed, the cause isn't always clear. But it's always worthwhile to try to find out the reason behind the delay, says reproductive endocrinologist and gynecologic surgeon Deborah Metzger, M.D., Ph.D., medical director of Helena Women's Health in San Jose, California, and medical advisor to this book.

A discussion with your doctor might reveal that you haven't been calculating ovulation correctly or are unknowingly using a lubricant with spermicide in it. There are lots of biological and environmental subtleties that make the difference between conceiving now or months later—or not at all. The subfertile woman may have one, rather than two, working ovaries. Subfertile men may have healthy sperm, but fewer of them. Such couples may eventually conceive naturally or, depending on how pressed for time they feel, may opt for medical interventions that can make conception more efficient.

Either way, it's essential to be evaluated. That way, couples who have more serious conditions, such as blocked fallopian tubes or the inability to produce sperm, won't spend time waiting for the impossible when they need medical procedures or alternative parenting plans, says Steven Sondheimer, M.D., professor of obstetrics and gynecology at the University of Pennsylvania Medical Center in Philadelphia and a spokesperson for the Association of Reproductive Health Professionals (ARHP).

Although many insurance carriers and medical textbooks advise couples to give themselves a year to conceive before seeing a doctor, it's more than fine to consult with a doctor before then if you are concerned, Dr. Sondheimer says. In fact, if any of the following are true for you or your mate, you should consult an infertility expert right away because you have a good chance of being subfertile.

* You miss periods, or your periods are less than 25 or more than 35 days apart

* You haven't conceived after 6 months of trying, and you are 35 or older (your husband's age is less important)

* Either of you has had chemotherapy

* Your mate suffered severe testicular trauma because of a sports injury or other accident or has had a testicle removed, undescended testes, childhood mumps, or another potentially sperm-compromising condition

* Either of you has had pelvic surgery, such as an appendectomy

* You have had a previous ectopic pregnancy

* You or your partner has any history of infection in the pelvic organs, such as chlamydia or pelvic inflammatory disease (PID)

* You or your partner has a chronic disease such as diabetes, high blood pressure, lupus, or kidney disease

THE INFERTILITY WORKUP

Getting to the bottom of fertility problems starts with your doc taking a thorough medical history of both you and your mate. Women should bring as much information as they have about their menstrual cycle patterns, including basal body temperature charts or other ovulation-tracking results. Both partners should be prepared to discuss previous childbearing experiences, sexual habits, any genetic conditions in the family, and their history of sexually transmitted diseases and other past infections and diseases.

Both partners will be given a standard physical, usually on the first or second visit. A woman's physical may include a Pap test and her first round of lab tests (if it's the right time in her cycle). The man's genitalia will be checked for any abnormalities, and he will give his first semen sample for analysis. (The basic workup requires two to three samples taken 1 month apart.)

An initial fertility evaluation, and your first round of tests, can be started with a primary care physician, obstetrician/gynecologist, or urologist. But it's advisable to escalate to an infertility specialist if you haven't conceived or gotten any answers after 3 months of treatment under the care of a primary physician.

Reproductive endocrinologists are obstetrician/gynecologists who have completed 2 additional years of study and research in treating reproductive disorders over and above standard obstetrics and gynecology training. They are considered definitive infertility specialists. Gynecologists, urologists, and other practitioners who devote their practice exclusively to infertility can also be considered specialists, according to the ARHP.

A complete infertility workup takes about 3 months, because sperm quality and monthly hormone changes need to be followed over a period of time. By the time all is said and done, your doctor should have checked four main elements: the number and quality of sperm, the maturation and release of your eggs, barriers to fertilization, and barriers to implantation and maintenance of pregnancy.

Screenings for Ovulatory Disorders

A woman's baby-making factory is essentially shut down, at least temporarily, if she's not releasing a monthly egg. If that egg is released at the wrong time, or when it's not fully formed, the factory's product won't pass inspection (fertilization and implantation). Production is also halted when a full staff of workers (in the form of ovulation-supporting hormones) don't show up for a shift or can't cooperate with other workers anywhere along the line.

Hormone imbalances that compromise egg development, release, fertilization, or implantation are *ovulatory disorders* of some kind. Ovulatory factors are the most common cause of infertility in women. Less commonly, ovulation is impeded by a physical abnormality, such as a benign tumor on the adrenal or pituitary gland, or congenitally malformed reproductive organs. But usually, ovulatory disorders are endocrine-related—and a series of lab tests can offer clues about how to resolve the problem.

In addition to considering the levels of individual reproductive hormones, doctors will also look at the relationships among those hormones. For example, polycystic ovary syndrome (PCOS), also known as Stein–Leventhal disease, is characterized by a pattern of deficient follicle-stimulating hormone (FSH) and progesterone levels, along with increased levels of testosterone, estrogen, and luteinizing hormone (LH). Another disorder, known as luteal phase defect (in which an egg can't implant or miscarries), usually shows inadequate postovulation progesterone levels but normal estrogen levels at midcycle.

Along with studying reproductive hormones, doctors will draw blood to test levels of thyroid and prolactin hormones. Over time, abnormal levels of these hormones can throw off the actual reproductive hormones, or they can cause fertility problems themselves, explains Eric Daiter, M.D., a reproductive endocrinologist in Edison, New Jersey. (See chapter 16 for more on hormone imbalances.)

While infertility specialists may vary somewhat in their protocols, most infertility workups include these basic lab tests, which may be coordinated with same-day ultrasounds.

* Labwork #1, done before ovulation, on day 2 or 3 of your cycle: baseline LH to FSH ratio, as well as estradiol

* Labwork #2, done 7 days after ovulation: progesterone, estradiol, prolactin, thyroid hormones (free T3, free T4), and thyroid-stimulating hormone (TSH) and, when indicated, an "androgen panel" (dehydroepiandrosterone sulfate [DHEAS], testosterone, androstenedione)

* Labwork #3, done midcycle: LH, FSH, estradiol, progesterone

Other possible lab tests in addition to the basic workup include:

* Clomiphene citrate challenge test: blood test done after a dosage of ovulation-inducing medication (clomiphene citrate, or Clomid) to see if poorly responding ovaries can be stimulated with medication

* Inhibin B: a protein made by the cells surrounding the eggs, measured as an indicator of ovarian reserve for women close to menopause

* Insulin levels: blood test done after drinking a special glucose-containing drink when PCOS or diabetes is suspected; recommended for all women over 35

* Postcoital test: sample of cervical fluid taken between 1 and 18 hours after intercourse during the ovulatory window to determine if a sperm can penetrate and survive in a woman's reproductive tract

* Endometrial biopsy: a small sample of the lining of the uterus taken to confirm whether and when ovulation occurred

Examining Your "Nest"

If an egg is the raw material in a woman's baby-making factory, her ovaries, fallopian tubes, and uterus are the basic machinery needed for re-

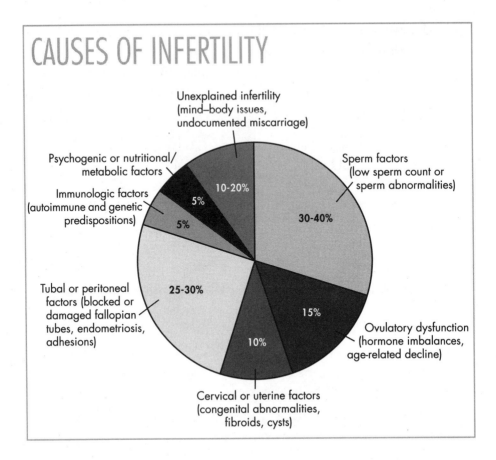

CAUSES OF INFERTILITY

Unexplained infertility (mind–body issues, undocumented miscarriage) 10-20%

Psychogenic or nutritional/metabolic factors 5%

Immunologic factors (autoimmune and genetic predispositions) 5%

Sperm factors (low sperm count or sperm abnormalities) 30-40%

Tubal or peritoneal factors (blocked or damaged fallopian tubes, endometriosis, adhesions) 25-30%

Ovulatory dysfunction (hormone imbalances, age-related decline) 15%

Cervical or uterine factors (congenital abnormalities, fibroids, cysts) 10%

production. In more organic terms, the stork can only make deliveries to accessible, safe "nests." Malfunctioning machinery—or structurally unsound nests—account for close to 40 percent of female infertility.

Some abnormalities have been present since birth and remain unrecognized until a woman experiences infertility. Similarly, an infection or injury sustained years ago could have created scar tissue that cements a woman's fallopian tubes shut or makes for an unfriendly lining of the uterus.

"Fibroids, cysts, polyps, or endometrial tissue implants in and around your uterus can potentially play the same role of an IUD [intrauterine device] contraceptive by getting in the way of an egg on its way to implantation," says Dr. Metzger. Later, fibroids and other tissue overgrowths could also crowd out a fetus. Sensitive images of their size and placement can be taken to determine if they could interfere with reproduction. (Read more about these structural problems in chapter 17.)

For the first level of structural tests, your doctor will want to know if your fallopian tubes are open and if your uterus is the normal shape and size. Any outstanding features like uterine fibroids or ovarian cysts will also be observed. If problems are found, you will most likely have a second level of tests to clarify the best treatment approach. Not only does this second level of tests give more sophisticated images of your reproductive organs, but it offers an opportunity to actually correct problems on the spot. If surgery is not an option to repair the abnormalities, an infertility specialist will usually recommend specific assisted reproductive techniques (ARTs) that can bypass the problem. (See chapter 17 for other options for resolving structural problems.)

These are the basic tests.

First Level:

* *Hysterosalpingography (HSG):* An x-ray shows the interior of the uterus and fallopian tubes after dye is pumped in through the cervix. This diagnostic test can also be therapeutic, since the liquid dye flushing through the tubes may clear a potential blockage.

* *Transvaginal ultrasound:* A sound wave device is inserted into the vagina to produce images of the uterus and ovaries. If fibroids or polyps are suspected, sterile water or saline is injected into the uterus for more sensitive imaging.

Second Level:

* *Hysteroscopy:* The inside of the uterus is viewed through a hysteroscope, a thin telescope-like device inserted through the cervix. This procedure may also include taking a tissue sample or making minor repairs, such as removing scar tissue.

* *Laparoscopy:* While the hysteroscope views the interior of the uterus, a laparoscope gives access to the exterior portion of the uterus, fallopian tubes, and ovaries. The telescope-like device is

inserted near the navel under general anesthesia. At this time, a skilled pelvic surgeon can "rebuild" tubes, remove growths, significantly reduce endometriosis, or collect precise information for future medical interventions.

INFERTILITY IS AN EQUAL-OPPORTUNITY CONDITION

Since half of all documented causes of infertility are related to men, it's just as important for your partner to seek evaluation and treatment as it is for you. Doctors stress complete couples care, since historical precedent places the responsibility for infertility disproportionately on women. For instance, despite being the "father" of our country, George Washington never grasped that he couldn't biologically father a child. The first president of the United States declared his wife Martha "barren" even though she bore four children in a previous marriage—unlike George, whose case of smallpox may well have rendered him sterile. Similarly, Middle Eastern kings who couldn't reproduce were known to send their entire harem to the doctor but never seek medical treatment themselves.

Pride or fear can prevent a guy from joining his wife at infertility evaluations, but in all fairness, men may also be misled, says Dr. Sondheimer. "Women will know they haven't ovulated if they skipped a menstrual cycle, but men don't have clear markers for their fertility. They assume that just because they ejaculate, viable sperm are present. However, there could be no sperm at all, low sperm concentrations, or abnormal sperm, no matter what volume of semen is produced," he says.

"There's no reason to leave it to chance, since semen analysis is quick, painless, and can save lots of heartache, time, and money," adds Philip Werthman, M.D., a urologist specializing in male infertility and microsurgery who is the director of the Center for Male Reproductive Medicine and chief of urology at Center City Hospital, both in Los Angeles. "Even *before* the woman starts her first workup, I usually recommend that her husband have a semen analysis so they know where they are starting from."

THE "STAIRSTEP" APPROACH TO MALE FERTILITY PROBLEMS

While a host of factors can cause female infertility, male infertility is a lot more straightforward. Here's the basic approach to treatment, beginning with the least invasive method and working up to progressively more complicated procedures.

1. Lifestyle modification. Lifestyle factors that could be compromising sperm are corrected. These could include nutritional deficiencies, excessive heat, hard bicycle seats, toxic chemicals, or substance abuse.

2. Medical problems. Every measure is taken to resolve genitourinary infections such as prostatitis and epididymitis. Structural problems like varicoceles or an obstructed epididymis can often be surgically treated so that the quality of sperm improves sufficiently, says Philip Werthman, M.D., a urologist specializing in male infertility and microsurgery and director of the Center for Male Reproductive Medicine in Los Angeles.

3. Hormone improvements. Clomiphene citrate, or Clomid (more commonly used for egg production), can stimulate the testicles to produce more sperm and testosterone. Medications can also be used to correct specific imbalances such as high prolactin levels.

4. Intrauterine insemination (IUI). Some men with low sperm counts could be potentially fertile if more of their sperm could reach the fallopian tubes with the help of insemination.

5. Intracytoplasmic sperm injection (ICSI). Even very low sperm count can often be overcome by directly inserting the sperm into the egg. In fact, half of men with *no* sperm in their semen will have some in their epididymides (the tubes where the sperm mature) or testes, which can be retrieved through a procedure known as needle aspiration. If no sperm are found, they still may possibly be retrieved by removing a bit of the sperm-generating tissue from the inside of the testicle.

6. Donor sperm. This is the last resort when the options listed above have produced no success. It is also recommended for men who have no sperm due to a mechanical blockage, congenital absence of sperm, or prior vasectomy.

A guy even has options of how he provides his specimen. The standard method is via masturbation at the doctor's office. If the idea of unlocked exam rooms gives your partner the heebie-jeebies, he can collect the sample at home through masturbation or with your help. For men who have difficulty masturbating or find the process ethically unacceptable, the doctor can provide a special condom to collect a specimen during intercourse.

Of course, a woman isn't advised to discontinue her evaluation and treatment plan even if her partner has been diagnosed with a sperm deficiency. Twenty-five percent of infertile couples have both male and female factors that contribute to the problem, according to the American Society for Reproductive Medicine.

THE LOW-TECH APPROACH TO INFERTILITY

Just as a forest is a dynamic, living organism of interrelated plants, insects, streams, and bacteria—rather than simply a cluster of trees—a reproductive system is more than a uterus and ovaries or testicles. A natural, "low-tech" approach to infertility considers the inability to conceive as a multisystem imbalance. Creativity, gentle nurturing, and lots of individual attention are put into restoring the health and balance of your body.

"Think about it. If you are looking for a place to live for 9 months, you aren't going to pick a slum. An embryo and fetus need a friendly, healthy environment," says Janet Zand, L.Ac., N.D., O.M.D., a doctor of naturopathy and doctor of oriental medicine in Austin, Texas, and coauthor of *Smart Medicine for Healthier Living*.

To create this type of environment, "we might have to peel off layers of toxicity, hormone disorders, allergies, emotional baggage, stress, chronic infections, and poor diets," says Serafina Corsello, M.D., executive administrator of the Wellness Medical Center of Integrative Medicine in New York City and author of *The Ageless Woman*. "A detailed, integrative medicine approach is worthwhile. Not only will it increase the body's inherent ability to conceive on its own, but creating a super immune system in the parents is key to having an exceptional child!"

An integrative medicine approach to infertility draws on the wisdom found in such unique but interrelated disciplines as bodywork, naturopathy, and Traditional Chinese Medicine. Each of these addresses specific concerns that could be upsetting the delicate balance of your reproductive system.

Bodywork. Structural imbalances that compromise fertility can be a result of poor posture and a sedentary lifestyle or an isolated injury like a fall off a bike or a car accident, says Nataly Pluta, P.T., A.Y.T., a physical therapist and yoga therapist who runs Pluta Movement Therapeutics in Del Mar, California. Physical therapists, massage therapists, yoga therapists, rolfers, and chiropractors all practice their own form of bodywork— "hands-on" therapy that can improve underlying, mechanical causes of infertility or enhance other treatments.

"Spinal malalignment and muscular imbalances can reduce the natural flow of the autonomic nervous system, which supplies the reproductive organs," Pluta explains. "In addition to aligning and stretching your spine and supporting structures, bodywork can also induce the relaxation response to help balance hormones."

Naturopathy. Nutrition-oriented practitioners may ask you to keep a food diary for a week so they can suggest better food choices and nutritional supplements tailored to your specific dietary shortcomings. "If a man or woman has been living on the 'standard American diet,' they are most likely deficient in several nutrients needed for optimum health as well as fertility. And a deficiency in just *one* key nutrient can impair a man or woman's fertility," says Ellen Kamhi, Ph.D., R.N., a health educator and practitioner based in Oyster Bay, New York, who is known as The Natural Nurse. She is the author of *Cycles of Life: Herbs and Energy Techniques for the Stages of a Woman's Life.*

"Reducing caffeine, eating unprocessed foods, reducing alcohol, getting off unnecessary medication—these things an infertility specialist will tell you, but a naturopathic doctor will tell you twice," comments Dr. Zand. Naturopathic physicians are graduates of medical school, where they spent as much time studying the basic sciences as conventional medical practitioners. But their clinical training focuses on nondrug modalities such as therapeutic nutrition, botanical medicine, spinal manipulation, homeopathy, mind–body approaches, and hydrotherapy.

When specific fertility problems are found, natural health practitioners make every effort to employ treatments that increase the body's own healing mechanisms, rather than drugs that overrride symptoms, says Jill E. Stansbury, N.D., a naturopathic physician specializing in reproductive health in Battle Ground, Washington, and chair of the botanical medicine department at the National College of Naturopathic Medicine in Portland, Oregon.

Traditional Chinese Medicine (TCM). TCM's approach to infertility is very different from that of Western medicine. Rather than focusing on the sperm and the egg, tremendous attention is paid to the spleen, liver, and kidneys (the spleen because of its influences on the immune system and bloodflow to the uterus, the liver because of its role in hormone balance, and the kidneys because they're considered the body's source of sexual energy). Two people who have the same infertility diagnosis in Western medicine might be given very different treatments in TCM because treatment will be tailored to each person's "constitution"—his or her unique strengths and weaknesses on a physical, emotional, and energetic level.

"The fact that the infertility rate is only 3 percent in China but over 15 percent in the United States reflects how effectively TCM can optimize fertility," says Wei Liu, M.P.H., T.C.M.D., a doctor of Chinese medicine; clinical professor at the American Academy of Acupuncture and Oriental Medicine in Roseville, Minnesota; and author of *Chinese Medicine for Infertility*.

The foundation of TCM treatment is acupuncture, Chinese herbs, and dietary modifications on a highly personalized level. Practitioners emphasize that the therapies are natural, affordable, and safe.

"Many women do not need fertility drugs and medically assisted reproductive technologies, yet they go through months of physical and emotional agony, not to mention the financial burden," says Randine Lewis,

L.Ac., Ph.D., an oriental medicine doctor with special training in infertility who is director of the Eastern Harmony Acupuncture and Herbal Clinic in Houston. "Conventional Western medicine offers a bigger bang, but we liken this to putting a thumbtack in the wall with a sledgehammer. TCM will put the tack in the wall with a thumb."

DEVELOPING A REALISTIC TREATMENT PLAN

"The essence of a realistic treatment plan is one with boundaries," Dr. Metzger says. "Everyone has a limit to what they can put forth physically, emotionally, and financially and should consider these limitations up front."

Know what's *really* involved before you start on a "simple medication" that requires you to get two ultrasound procedures and take injections, doubles your chances of having triplets, and can increase your risk for cancer—all for a four-figure bill that your insurance doesn't pick up. Be fully informed about treatments in terms of time, money, stress, side effects, and other demands. Make sure you have plenty of literature that spells out the details, and talk to other infertility patients so you can make the decision that's right for you. "Don't let your treatment become a giant boulder heading for more and more demanding procedures if you or your partner isn't up for it," says Dr. Werthman.

"Communication is essential every step of the way," notes Dr. Sondheimer. Mapping out the next 6 months to a year of treatment with your partner and doctor gives you a greater sense of control. "Every month can seem like a lifetime when you can't conceive, so it's very therapeutic to know what's coming if one procedure doesn't work out," he says.

When you have a good plan, you'll see that there's a logical progression of treatment protocols that moves from the simplest to the most demanding physically and financially. Keep the following principles in mind as you go along.

Give interventions about three cycles. It may take three or four cycles for treatment to adequately address the cause of infertility. But after this

WHAT WORKED FOR US

SHE TOOK SWIFT ACTION AT THE FIRST SIGN OF MENOPAUSE

Kay Williams* knew that her mother had experienced premature menopause and that this increased her chances of following the same fate. Still, it didn't worry her enough to try to start a family before the age of 35. Although her menstrual cycles were slightly irregular, she had no trouble conceiving her first child at 36. But when the Boston social worker and her husband were thinking about a second child, Kay began to experience hot flashes.

Sure enough, a test measuring her levels of follicle-stimulating hormone (FSH) indicated that her ovaries were almost completely shut down at the age of 39—when most of her friends were just starting premenopause. A local fertility specialist told her nothing could be done. If she wanted another child, it would have to be through adoption or a donor egg. She sought another opinion, but "the second specialist was even more dismissive. He made me feel done for," Kay recalls.

"If I knew it was going to be like this, I don't think I would have waited so long to try for my pregnancies," she admits. Kay and her husband, a physician, agreed that they would be realistic but wanted to pursue limited infertility treatment. So she returned to the first infertility clinic and implored the doctor to give her clomiphene citrate (Clomid), which is used to stimulate egg production. To everyone's surprise, Kay produced two eggs, according to her ultrasound test. The next test revealed that the couple's sperm and egg had united. Kay was quickly given supplemental progesterone to discourage miscarriage. Miraculously, within just 3 months of that high FSH test result, Kay was pregnant.

To Kay, it all seems meant to be. She experienced no side effects from the medication, nor did she have any difficulties with pregnancy or childbirth. In fact, sometimes she wonders if she would have conceived anyway without the medication. But she and her husband know that it may have opened their narrow window of opportunity just a little wider. And their blond-haired, blue-eyed little boy proved their timely and proactive medical decisions infinitely worthwhile.

*Name has been changed for confidentiality

number of cycles of any treatment, the chances for success drop. A good treatment plan should recognize the law of diminishing returns. If no pregnancy has occurred within three or four cycles, reevaluate the situation and plan the next step, advises Dr. Metzger.

Budget for the end of the line. Two cycles of in vitro fertilization (IVF) can cost $20,000. When couples don't talk to their physicians about how much they've budgeted, or insurance pays only a certain amount, some physicians make the mistake of frittering away the entire budget on expensive testing and treatment and don't leave any to pay for alternatives.

Don't be too dazzled by high-tech procedures. Some infertility centers are quick to label someone's infertility "unexplained" and rush them into IVF or another major procedure. Other times, couples act rashly when they hear the biological clock ticking. "Take time to look for and treat underlying problems," stresses Dr. Werthman. "High-tech interventions are diminished anyway if your physical or emotional health is poor. Plus, fertility drugs and assisted reproduction aren't permanent solutions. If you want more children, you may need to go through the whole ordeal again."

Have a plan that alleviates stress rather than creating it. Attitude toward treatment can statistically alter success rates, according to University of California researchers. They found that women with increased anger, hostility, or depression had fewer embryos that transferred for IVF and gamete intrafallopian tube transfer (GIFT) procedures than the least depressed and hostile patients. And feelings of guilt about treatment were associated with slightly lower infant birth weights. And "for people who aren't using ART, stress and anxiety about infertility can interfere with the most important part of the picture—by keeping them from having intercourse," points out Dr. Sondheimer.

Make sure you're partnered with the right doctor. "A competent provider will shape the treatment to the needs of the patients, and not vice versa," says Dr. Metzger. RESOLVE: The National Infertility Association can refer you to more than 600 physicians who meet its high standards. Contact RESOLVE at (888) 623-0744 or www.resolve.org.

Quit while you're ahead. "With infertility treatment, knowing when to stop or move on is as difficult for the couple as it is for a gambler," says Dr. Metzger. "All too often, a couple can become like a gambler who continues to put his coins into the slot machine, thinking that the next one will surely be the jackpot. It is important to avoid emotional as well as finan-

(continued on page 232)

TAKE TECHNOLOGY WITH CAUTION

Before beginning any high-tech fertility treatment plan, be sure you have all the facts about its associated health risks. These may include:

Multiple births. To increase the chances of success, assisted reproductive procedures routinely transfer more than one fertilized egg. For many couples, a potentially overcrowded nursery seems like an easy choice over an empty one. But there are more serious considerations than the 1,000 diaper changes a month required for triplet newborns. Carrying more than one baby means a higher risk for pregnancy and delivery complications, including low birth weight, birth defects, preterm birth, and miscarriage. Twins are five times less likely and triplets are 13 times less likely than "singletons" to survive their first year of life.

Increased risk of birth defects. As the technology to treat infertility quickly advances, researchers are scrambling to analyze the impact it has on new generations of "high-tech babies." Worldwide, some troubling data have noted higher numbers of birth defects and impaired mental development in study groups of children conceived with in vitro fertilization (IVF) and intracytoplasmic sperm injection (ICSI). When British researchers analyzed the outcome of 100,454 Australian infants, they found that ICSI babies were *twice as likely* to have a major birth defect. In another study on 89 children born through assisted reproductive techniques, 17 percent of ICSI babies and 2 percent of children conceived through IVF experienced mental delay, compared to only 1 percent of the children conceived naturally.

"Antifertility" effects. Rather than helping nature along, certain side effects caused by fertility treatments can actually detract from the process on a physical or emotional level. For some women, fertility drugs can dry up cervical mucus—which is like knocking down the bridge that sperm needs to travel toward the egg. And the stress and regimentation of infertility treatments can spoil the urge to make love for many couples. Duke University psychologists in Durham, North Carolina, polled infertility patients and found that many women experienced less sexual arousal, had less sex, and were overall less satisfied with the quality of their sexual relationships as a result of treatment.

General health risks. Several studies have suggested that women who take ovulation-inducing drugs, especially women who use them but don't get pregnant, have a potentially increased risk of ovarian and breast tumors. And ART slightly raises the risk for ectopic pregnancy, in which the egg implants in the wrong place and can lead to a life-threatening hemorrhage.

The following chart compares the risks associated with each assisted reproduction method and is based on information compiled by the Centers for Disease Control and Prevention from 370 fertility clinics.

Method	Success Rates per Cycle	Miscarriage Rates	Multiple Birth Rates	Approximate Costs per Cycle
Natural conception	20%	15%–20%	1%	$15 ovulation test kit
Ovulation-inducing drugs	8%–10%	20%–50%	5%–10%	$80
Superovulation drugs	12%–30%	20%	20%	$800–$2,000 (including required ultrasound and lab work)
Intrauterine insemination (IUI)	5%–14%	20%	20%–30% if used with superovulation drugs	$800 plus the cost of fertility medications
In vitro fertilization (IVF)	25%	20%–25%	37%	$10,000 plus the cost of medications
Gamete intrafallopian transfer (GIFT)	24%	20%–25%	37%	$12,000 plus the cost of medications
Zygote intrafallopian tube transfer (ZIFT)	27%	20%–25%	37%	$12,000 plus the cost of medications
ICSI	32%	20%–25%	37%	$15,000 (including egg retrieval and insemination)

cial bankruptcy," she emphasizes. (For further information on moving on after stopping infertility treatment, see chapter 19.)

Fertility Medications

Fertility medications are like power surges to the ovaries that buzz them to wake up and release an egg. Even for ovaries that aren't "asleep," these surges can induce more regular timing of ovulation or make more eggs available for an ART procedure. The "entry level" fertility drug is clomiphene citrate (Clomid), which acts on the hypothalamus and pituitary gland to stimulate ovulation-regulating FSH and LH. If it works, the woman will ovulate 5 to 10 days after finishing a 5-day round of the drug. Typically, it is used for three to six cycles before trying something else.

The next treatment level is *superovulation*. Drugs known as menotropins or gonadotropins are used alone or combined with clomiphene citrate for an even bigger "surge." Gonadotropins supplement the actual hormones that trigger an egg to leave the ovary—either FSH or human menopausal gonadotropin (hMG). Human chorionic gonadotropin (hCG) is injected when an ultrasound test reveals that eggs have matured.

Fertility drugs can be so taxing to the ovaries that mild overstimulation is experienced by about 20 percent of women taking menotropins. Symptoms include abdominal pain, nausea, diarrhea, vomiting, ovarian cyst formation, and vision changes. A more serious effect is ovarian hyperstimulation syndrome (OHSS), which approximately 1 to 3 percent of women experience. OHSS requires hospitalization because it can cause kidney damage, blood clots, dehydration, or breathing difficulties.

Although they aren't officially fertility drugs, thyroid replacement, prolactin-lowering medications, and insulin-sensitizing agents might be prescribed if laboratory tests have revealed abnormal hormone levels. These drugs alone may correct anovulation or subfertility.

The "ART" of Assisted Reproduction

More than 70,000 babies have been born in the United States as a result of ART. As detailed below, there is a progression of ART techniques,

HIGH-TECH FERTILITY TREATMENT AND THE 35+ WOMAN

The commonly cited statistic is that 85 percent of couples conceive within their first year of trying. But in reality, the statistics are not as glowing for women over the age of 35. The Association of Reproductive Health Professionals reports that one-third of couples in which the female partner is 35 or older will have problems with fertility and two-thirds of women won't conceive without intervention by age 40.

Since the chances are high that you are going to seek treatment, the following advice is designed to help the 35+ woman navigate through the options.

* Always get a follicle-stimulating hormone (FSH) test on day 3 of your cycle. Don't assume that just because you have a period, you're ovulating.

* Consider getting the inhibin B test for more information about ovarian reserve.

* Get your 2-hour postglucose insulin levels tested. This is a common (and commonly missed) infertility factor in women over 35.

* Since you are likely to take clomiphene citrate (Clomid) to enhance ovulation, be certain to start it on day 2 or 3 of your cycle rather than day 5—it will lower the risk of miscarriage from 50 percent to 20 percent.

* Women over the age of 35 require more progesterone to maintain a pregnancy, so be sure your doctor writes you a prescription for either oral or vaginal progesterone.

* Be realistic when considering assisted reproductive techniques (ARTs). The reported 25 percent ART success rate is highly dependent on age. For 40-year-old women, the success rate for live births is actually 16 percent, and it drops to 3 percent for 43-year-old women. That's why many infertility clinics won't accept women over the age of 44 for treatment unless they agree to use a younger woman's egg.

* Consider whether adoption is a better choice for you. If, in your heart, what is really important to you is becoming a parent rather than creating a child who is biologically related to you, adoption may be an option you'll want to explore. The costs of adoption are similar to those of in vitro fertilization, but with adoption, you can spare yourself the possible heartache of failed attempts and miscarriage.

from those that help nature along to those that manipulate the entire conception process. A couple may opt to use donor egg or sperm for these ART techniques if their own aren't viable.

Insemination. Sperm is placed in a woman's vagina, cervix, or uterus by means other than intercourse. Ejaculated semen is processed to concentrate sperm into a very small volume of fluid. Most commonly, the fluid is placed in the uterus in a procedure called intrauterine insemination (IUI). IUI is used to overcome infertility associated with low sperm count, cervical mucus problems, and antisperm antibodies and for nonspecifically enhancing fertility.

Gamete intrafallopian transfer (GIFT). After a woman takes egg-stimulating medication, one or more of her eggs are removed from the ovary via laparoscope or by an ultrasound-guided needle. A mixture of egg and sperm is then placed in the fallopian tubes for fertilization to occur.

Zygote intrafallopian tube transfer (ZIFT). Eggs are obtained as in GIFT, mixed with sperm, and left to fertilize in a laboratory dish. Laparoscopy is used to insert the embryos into the fallopian tube the next day, where they are expected to travel into the uterus and implant.

IVF. In vitro fertilization, first used in 1981, is the most established of the embryo-transfer methods. Eggs are removed from the ovaries as in GIFT and ZIFT. They are given several days to be fertilized with "washed" sperm in the lab and are then placed directly into the woman's uterus using needles and a plastic catheter.

Intracytoplasmic sperm injection (ICSI). Technicians directly intervene in the fertility process by shooting ejaculated sperm into the eggs. If fertilization is successful, the eggs are placed in the woman's uterus to grow.

16

Natural Solutions for Hormone Disorders

When it comes to fertility drugs, one woman's miracle might be another's nightmare. For some, fertility drugs are just the boost their bodies need to trigger ovulation. But for Jane Baltimore (name has been changed for privacy), they produced nightmarish side effects, caused a lot of heartache—and weren't even necessary.

Although she was ovulating, Jane's doctor recommended she take clomiphene citrate (Clomid) to normalize her cycles, which were between 36 and 45 days long. "During my treatment, I experienced hot flashes, dizziness, and mood swings. After seven cycles and three inseminations with no pregnancy, I insisted we stop the drug," Jane recalls.

The next fertility specialist she saw gave her egg-releasing hormone injections with the drug Lupron. Even more overwhelming side effects, including an abnormally rapid heart rate, debilitating headaches, and fatigue, sent Jane to the hospital. "I was treated as a psychiatric patient," she remembers. The only thing that was crazy, Jane contends, was the overload of synthetic hormones that doctors used to treat her alleged infertility instead of paying attention to her overall health.

When Jane got out of the hospital, she consulted a natural health practitioner, who put more faith in vitamins than drugs. Jane filled out a long questionnaire to evaluate her diet, lifestyle, and emotional health—things that nobody ever asked her about before. She was given tests for such conditions as liver toxicity and hidden allergies. Her "prescription" included infusions of vitamins and minerals, a vegetarian diet, bowel cleansing, and stress reduction through biofeedback.

Jane's cycles snapped back into clockwork, 30- to 31-day patterns that she hadn't experienced for several years. "Everyone I knew told me that I looked fabulous and exuded energy and vitality," she says. As it turns out, Jane became pregnant naturally and had a baby boy with "perfect 10" Apgar scores (an obstetrical rating for newborn health).

Fertility drugs are not for everyone. Some women have to stop taking them because their ovaries have become hyperstimulated (a life-threatening condition) or they've developed cysts. Others are disenchanted with the statistics on their use, such as the 50 percent rate of miscarriage with Clomid or the elevated chances of multiple births (20 percent for menotropins). Fortunately, for women who can't take fertility drugs or who opt to not contend with the potential risks and side effects, there are alternatives.

It's difficult to compare the success rates of fertility drugs with the protocols of natural health practitioners because practically no clinical studies have been done. In one preliminary trial that observed 96 women who took a combination of homeopathic remedies and a leading fertility herb, success rates were similar to those seen with fertility drugs. But it's really comparing apples with oranges—or an apple with a whole bowl of assorted fruit. Natural therapies strive not only to improve fertility but to restore the overall functioning of the endocrine system and its support team, including the immune and nervous systems, explains Jill E. Stansbury, N.D., a naturopathic physician specializing in reproductive health in Battle Ground, Washington, and chair of the botanical medicine department at the National College of Naturopathic Medicine in Portland, Oregon.

START WITH DETOXIFICATION

Modern living isn't easy on our body's detoxification system. We bombard it with pollution, medications, alcohol, hormone-laced meat and dairy products, pesticides, and the artificial colors, flavors, preservatives, and other laboratory-concocted ingredients that make up highly processed foods.

"Think of the body's detoxification system as a pool filter. When more junk comes through than it's designed to process, it overflows," says Ellen Kamhi, Ph.D., R.N., a health educator and practitioner based in Oyster Bay, New York, who is known as The Natural Nurse. She is the author of *Cycles of Life: Herbs and Energy Techniques for the Stages of a Woman's Life.*

The liver, kidney, skin, and bowels are the main organs that make up the detoxification system. In addition, the lymph nodes serve as minifilters in various locations, such as the armpits, groin, and throat. One of the liver's main responsibilities is to break down hormones, including 40 different varieties of estrogens found both in our bodies and in our environment, says Dr. Kamhi. Throw in too many other odd jobs, and it's like expecting the pool filter to clear out leaves and dirt plus a tank of tar.

A bogged-down detoxification system can lead to several hormone imbalances. "When a woman has a luteal phase defect (miscarriage or implantation problems related to irregular progesterone and estrogen levels), one of the first things I consider is suboptimal liver function," says Dr. Stansbury. In a man, sperm count and sperm quality can also be affected by the liver.

"If a woman comes to me with infertility, detoxification is always the first line of defense. I recommend she stays on birth control and does a detoxification for 3 months before starting on any specific therapies," explains Dr. Kamhi. "Detoxification makes the lymph fluid less viscous [thick], allowing it to flow more easily throughout all body tissues."

Top infertility doctors have sought out Dr. Kamhi to help with female clients who haven't had success even after several rounds of in vitro fertilization (IVF). The detoxification tips that follow are what she recommends to them and to hundreds of other couples who have gone on to conceive.

Try a minifast. Fasting is a method widely recognized throughout history to rest and heal the body. It's not necessary to "starve" to accomplish your goal. Dr. Kamhi's minifast allows you to eat as much of a nourishing soup (see "Slurp Some Soup to Detoxify Your Body") and drink as much puri-

SLURP SOME SOUP TO DETOXIFY YOUR BODY

The following vitamin-packed soup can be eaten during a detoxifying minifast, says Ellen Kamhi, Ph.D., R.N., a health educator and practitioner based in Oyster Bay, New York, who is known as The Natural Nurse. She is the author of *Cycles of Life: Herbs and Energy Techniques for the Stages of a Woman's Life.* Feel free to consume as much of the soup as you'd like, along with plenty of purified water.

You can purchase nori sea vegetable and Bragg Liquid Aminos at health food stores. The aminos can also be ordered from the company's Web site, www.bragg.com.

Detoxifying Vegetable Soup

1	organic onion, cut into wedges
1	head organic cabbage, sliced
2	cloves organic garlic, sliced
2	organic carrots, sliced
2	organic celery ribs, sliced
1	bunch parsley
5	organic kale leaves
2	sheets nori sea vegetable
4	pieces organic okra
1	cup organic brown rice
	Bragg Liquid Aminos, to taste
2	quarts filtered water

In a large pot, combine the onion, cabbage, garlic, carrots, celery, parsley, kale, nori sea vegetable, okra, rice, liquid aminos, and water. Simmer for 1½ hours.

fied water as you want for 3 days. Any two organic fruits can be included as snacks, too. If you feel light-headed, you can also have a high-protein drink. (Plain whey is best.) For maximum effect, continue past the 3 days for up to 7 days, says Dr. Kamhi. She recommends that the minifast be done once a season. When you end your minifast, eat no fried, processed, or sugar-laden foods for at least another 2 days, Dr. Kamhi says. "Of course, avoiding these foods altogether is the best choice," she notes.

Cleanse your colon. If you are constipated or have gone about 24 hours without having a bowel movement, work psyllium into your detoxification protocol. Dr. Kamhi recommends ¼ teaspoon of psyllium seeds in 8 ounces of water two times per day. You may also find it helpful to use an enema during detoxification, particularly if you're constipated, she says. Once you are regular for several days (at least one, unstrained movement every day), you can phase out the psyllium.

Empower your liver with herbs. Although it's more common to think of "fertility herbs" as those that have direct hormone-like effects, the real powerhouse herbs are those that allow your body to correct its own imbalances. Any liver-supporting herb fills the bill, including dandelion, burdock, and milk thistle. Combine liquid extracts of the three herbs (two parts dandelion, one part burdock, and one part milk thistle), and take 4 milliliters (about 1 teaspoon) of the mixture twice a day. You can put the herbs in water or juice to dilute their intense flavor.

Enhance your lymph nodes. "You'll know your lymph nodes are being cleared if they feel a little tender," says Dr. Kamhi. "The discomfort will last only a few days."

"To help your lymph fluid do its job, take the herb cleavers, in 2-milliliter doses (about ½ teaspoon) of liquid extract, twice a day," recommends Dr. Kamhi. "You know it's working if you urinate a lot, since cleavers has diuretic properties."

Exfoliate from the outside in. A technique called "dry brushing" stimulates the lymphatic system and also removes dead skin cells. Purchase a dry skin brush or a bath brush made of soft natural bristles, such as sisal, or a loofah sponge. These items can be found in health food stores and some drugstores. Before getting into the shower or bath, brush your skin with long strokes toward your heart, using enough pressure to feel some light friction.

Jump away toxins. Purchase a minitrampoline and place it where you will see it and won't be able to resist the daily urge to rebound, suggests Dr. Kamhi. Not only does trampoline jumping indulge your playful spirit, but it is highly effective at stimulating a sluggish lymphatic system. "I always include it in the protocol for women with fibroid and cystic conditions," she says. Bonuses are that it boosts your heart rate and decreases cellulite!

Treat yourself to a monthly massage. A full-body, deep-tissue massage every 3 weeks can do wonders for detoxification and circulation. If you can't afford a professional, get into the habit of sharing massages with your friends and family when you get together. "I've gotten my kids well-trained to give good massages," Dr. Kamhi relates.

NORMALIZE YOUR MONTHLY CYCLES

A woman's monthly reproductive hormone rhythms can be fickle. Intercontinental air travel, strenuous exercise, sudden weight loss, or the emotional intensity of a death in the family or a career change are just a few of the experiences that can bring on your period at the wrong time or stifle ovulation for a month or two. An in-depth discussion with an infertility specialist or natural health practitioner can help identify anything you might be doing that could be disrupting the hormonal rhythms that control ovulation.

When menstrual cycles are shorter than 25 or longer than 35 days, it's essential to have a complete workup to make sure there's no major medical cause, such as lesions on the pituitary gland, insulin resistance, or premature menopause, cautions reproductive endocrinologist and gynecologic surgeon Deborah Metzger, M.D., Ph.D., medical director of Helena Women's Health in San Jose, California, and medical advisor to this book.

Standard infertility blood tests can also pick up a distinct pattern of hormone imbalance that indicates polycystic ovary syndrome (PCOS), otherwise known as Stein–Leventhal disease. This disorder is characterized by increased levels of insulin that signal the ovaries to produce an excess of androgen (male hormones) and estrogen. The overworked ovaries often bubble up with cysts but do not produce mature eggs.

Women with PCOS are given the option of several medications to restore their egg-creating capacities. Eighty percent of nonovulating women with PCOS will ovulate with the use of the fertility drug clomiphene citrate (Clomid). But it might not be necessary to resort to fertility drugs.

"Medications that lower insulin levels, such as Glucophage (metformin hydrochloride) and Avandia (rosiglitazone maleate), can regulate the menstrual cycle and improve ovulation as well as clomiphene can," says Dr. Metzger. In fact, even women who don't have all the signs and symptoms of PCOS may benefit, she points out. "Insulin treatment is often the boost needed for women with unexplained infertility or women over the age of 35. I can't even count all the women I've seen who couldn't get pregnant after several rounds of IVF, and ended up having high insulin levels. We put them on Glucophage, and they conceived on their own," says Dr. Metzger.

Of course, it's important to complement drug treatment with an insulin-modifying diet, which was discussed in chapter 3. In addition, daily exercise and weight loss (if you're overweight) help increase the sensitivity of cells to insulin and can help your body restore normal ovary function.

After any specific lifestyle or medical factors like PCOS are corrected— or if none can be identified—try the following additional tips to foster cycle regularity.

Take a night-light prescription. As we discussed in chapter 14, researchers at the University of California, San Diego, Sleep Lab were able to alter the length of women's menstrual cycles by exposing them to a night-light in the middle of their cycles, while they slept. In fact, women whose cycles were abnormally long (an average of 45 days) got closer to a more consistent 33-day pattern during the study. "Two previously infertile women even became pregnant during these light experiments," says Daniel Kripke, M.D., world-famous circadian rhythm expert, professor of psychiatry at the university, and current director of the lab. One theory as to why the women's cycles evened out is that the light decreased blood levels of mela-tonin, a brain chemical that is usually elevated in women with suppressed ovulation. "Whatever the case, there's no harm in women with long cycles or luteal phase defects trying the protocol at home," Dr. Kripke says. All you need is a lamp with a 100-watt bulb placed about a yard from your pillow. Turn it on about a half-hour before going to bed, and turn it off when you wake in the morning. Do this during days 13 to 17 of your cycle (starting 13 days after the first day of your period).

Use a simple reflexology technique. Reflexology—the stimulation of trigger points on the foot and ankle—is another natural health method that can gently support hormone balance. Dr. Kamhi teaches it to all her infertility patients. "I have definitely seen it bring on women's periods that were pre-viously out of sync," says Dr. Kamhi. "That doesn't mean that it is dra-matic enough to dislodge a fetus if a woman does get pregnant, but I do recommend doing it more gently after the time of ovulation," she says.

REFLEXOLOGY FOR HORMONE BALANCE

To encourage the timely arrival of your period, help a partner locate the tender spots between your heel and ankle bone on both sides of your foot. Have him use a fingertip from each hand to simultaneously rub these trigger points in a clockwise motion on one side and a counter-clockwise motion on the other.

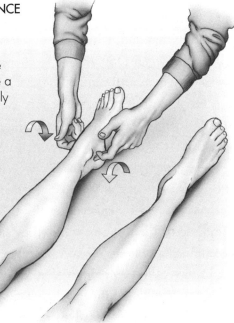

You can find the trigger points for the ovaries and uterus by feeling around for tender spots on either side of the ankle. They are in a small indentation between the heel and the ankle bone. It's best to ask a partner for help so you don't have to bend your knee and disrupt the flow to the neurological system. To encourage your period at the right time, rub hard in a clockwise motion on one side while you simultaneously rub counterclockwise on the opposite side. (You can really stimulate those points by using two pencil erasers.) If you are actively trying to get pregnant, rub only to the point of tenderness, not pain, which you'd do to bring on a cycle.

Try the vitex solution. The herb vitex agnus-castus, also called chaste tree, is the closest thing to clomiphene citrate (without the side effects) in Mother Nature's medicine chest. That's because it enhances ovulation by acting directly on the hypothalamus and the pituitary gland to stimulate the chain reaction of hormones that releases an egg. Vitex has such a normalizing effect on hormone rhythms that it can restore periods in women with no menstruation at all, Dr. Stansbury says. It is recommended for women whose cycles are disrupted because of low progesterone levels, high prolactin levels, or excess estrogen. Dr. Stansbury prescribes 1 to 3 teaspoons a day, as a tincture.

Caution: Vitex should not be taken with dopamine-receptor antagonist drugs, such as olanzapine (Zyprexa) or risperidone (Risperdal), or with any other fertility drugs or prescription hormone therapies, because it has similar effects. Note that during the first month of treatment, the length of your cycle may temporarily shorten or lengthen before stabilizing. Most women notice normalization within two menstrual cycles, and after 6 months to a year, vitex produces permanent results. Stop taking it after 6 to 8 months or once you are pregnant.

Don't overuse nonsteroidal anti-inflammatory drugs (NSAIDs). "The physical release of an egg from the ovary seems to be partly dependent upon a class of molecules called prostaglandins. Nonsteroidal anti-inflammatory medications such as Aleve and Motrin block prostaglandins, and therefore may interfere with ovulation," says Eric Daiter, M.D., a reproductive endocrinologist in Edison, New Jersey. Try not to use them starting several days prior to ovulation, he advises.

Resolve anemia. Do you have irregular periods, find yourself often weak and fatigued, and bruise easily? Women who are anemic may stop menstruating as their bodies attempt to avoid the loss of iron. Ask your practitioner about blood tests and treatment for anemia, recommends Dr. Stansbury.

KEEP SUGAR AND YEAST UNDER CONTROL

Sugar decreases the body's overall immune function. For instance, a high-sugar diet can deplete many of the nutrients that are essential to fertility, and it can cause B vitamins to have trouble penetrating the white blood cells, says Dr. Metzger.

"By sugar, I mean anything that elevates insulin levels, including refined flour products, beer, caffeine, and sweeteners like honey, corn syrup, and table sugar," Dr. Metzger explains. Some women's insulin levels go so high in response to sugar and refined carbohydrates that they stop ovulating. This includes women with blatant insulin-sensitive conditions like PCOS and diabetes, but they aren't the only ones who need to put the brakes on sugar. Sugar has detrimental effects on egg development in the ovaries—for every woman. High-sugar diets also impair sperm motility and promote the growth of yeast in the body, a common but often unrecognized infertility factor.

Candidiasis is a condition that results from the overgrowth of the yeast-like *Candida albicans* fungus, explains Wei Liu, M.P.H., T.C.M.D., a doctor of Chinese medicine; clinical professor at the American Academy of Acupuncture and Oriental Medicine in Roseville, Minnesota; and author of *Chinese Medicine for Infertility*. "*Candida* are part of the normal flora of our bodies found in the mouth, vagina, intestines, and other organs, but a disproportionate amount of *Candida albicans* can lead to a compromised digestive system, immune system, and hormone system," she says. We create the environment for yeast overgrowth by consuming a lot of sugar, yeast, and alcohol. Also, antibiotics wipe out beneficial bacteria that help keep *Candida* under control.

During their metabolic process, *Candida* release estrogen-like compounds that can encourage estrogen dominance and related hormone imbalances, such as luteal phase defect, says Dr. Kamhi. Yeast infections can be passed back and forth between partners during intercourse and can prevent sperm from entering the uterus. An imbalance of yeast and bacteria in the bowels causes "intestinal dysbiosis," which is often the underlying cause of irritable bowel symptoms, food allergies, and poor absorption of those fertility-necessary nutrients, adds Dr. Metzger.

Candidiasis is also a threat to fertility because the body may release anti-*Candida* antibodies in an attempt to clear the imbalance, which could potentially create an autoimmune response that could attack an egg or sperm, adds Dr. Kamhi.

"Candidiasis is an aggressive condition that needs to be aggressively treated," says Dr. Liu. "It's worthwhile to consult a natural health practitioner to help you get it under control."

Taming candidiasis may take a lot of discipline. But in addition to getting a fertility boost, you'll relieve candidiasis-related symptoms, including abdominal bloating, skin fungal conditions and rashes, chronic fatigue, poor memory and concentration, headaches, sugar cravings, and genital itching. Here is the program to knock out this multisystem imbalance.

Step 1: Fight off yeast overgrowth with an antifungal remedy. Options include the drug nystatin; herbal remedies such as pau d'arco, caprylic acid, uva ursi, grapeseed extract, oil of oregano, and garlic; or the Chinese formulas coptis and Long Dan Xie Gan Wan.

Step 2: Eliminate *all* yeast-based and fermented products from your diet. These include yeast-based breads, crackers, and pretzels; beer and other alcoholic beverages; cheese, vinegar, and pickled products; mushrooms; soy sauce, miso, and tempeh; yeast-treated canned goods like soup; and even yeast-based nutritional supplements. Doctors advise their patients to stay off these until they have experienced yeast die-off, which can take between 1 and 3 months.

Step 3: Cut way back on sugar. All simple carbohydrates feed *Candida*. That means you'll need to avoid all "white foods"—wheat-based baked goods, white pasta, commercial cereal, potatoes, and table sugar, says Dr. Metzger. The commercial sweetener Splenda and the herbal sweetener stevia are permitted, however, since they don't have the same effects on blood sugar, she says.

Step 4: Take a daily "probiotic" supplement. Hundreds of different microorganisms, or flora, live in your gastrointestinal tract. Because of their roles in digestion, nutrient absorption, and immune support, many of these microorganisms are considered "friendly flora," or beneficial bacteria. When their populations are high enough, probiotics also prevent the overproliferation of *Candida*. That's why experts recommend you take bioactive nutrients like acidophilus and bifidus. They are available at health food stores in freeze-dried capsules or in their active form as capsules, loose powder, or liquid (which can be found in the refrigerator section). While fermented dairy products are a traditional source of beneficial bacteria, different brands of yogurt vary in their bacteria strain and potency—in fact, some have no active cultures or defeat the yeast-clobbering purpose if they are sweetened. Some popular probiotic brands include Solgar, Nature's Plus, and Nature's Way. Purchase a product that says it contains at least 5 billion active cultures, and follow package directions. In addition, taking a *pre*biotic such as whey (either formulated in your probiotic or as a separate supplement) really helps the *pro*biotics to establish themselves and multiply in the body.

TREATING SPECIFIC IMBALANCES

When glaring hormone imbalances are picked up on a laboratory test for infertility, drugs are prescribed to increase or decrease the levels of individual hormones or to override the imbalance. Experts acknowledge, however, that not all hormone imbalances are picked up on conventional tests. For one thing, labs tests don't flag subclinical hormone imbalances—levels just outside of what's abnormal. Yet not only are subclinical levels often enough to cause fertility problems, but they may be precursors to more serious imbalances.

For example, subclinical hypothyroidism may interfere with fertility by lowering libido or causing irregular ovulation. Plus, it's essential to detect even subtle thyroid imbalances because the demands of pregnancy require much more thyroid hormone than a woman usually needs. Insufficient thyroid levels during pregnancy can lead to fetal growth retardation and miscarriage, says Dr. Daiter.

The fact is, hormone levels have some individual variability, so what's normal for one woman may produce antifertility symptoms for another woman, says Randine Lewis, L.Ac., Ph.D., an oriental medicine doctor with special training in infertility who is director of the Eastern Harmony Acupuncture and Herbal Clinic in Houston. In addition, if some tests aren't timed correctly, the imbalance won't be caught, Dr. Lewis says. "Progesterone deficiency is probably missed more than anything else because they test it only on day 21 of a woman's cycle, even if the woman ovulates on a different schedule," she says. "If a woman falls within normal range on day 21, she's not considered to have a luteal phase defect." Dr. Lewis's experience has led her to believe that even women with an apparently normal test result can have low progesterone levels. "It's not necessarily a strict progesterone deficiency anyway," she says. "It may be that the estrogen receptors aren't primed within the endometrium."

The following advice offers general hormone-balancing strategies that can help resolve deficiencies that might not be detected during regular testing. It includes steps to improve overall endocrine health and some nondrug options to support individual hormones.

Boosting Progesterone

Low progesterone is associated with luteal phase defect, in which the uterine lining isn't adequately prepared to support implantation. Low levels of progesterone are also a prime cause of miscarriage. A German study found low progesterone (coupled with increased prolactin) to be a cause of infertility in 62 percent of 753 infertile women. One indication of low progesterone is severe PMS, notes Serafina Corsello, M.D., executive administrator of the Wellness Medical Center of Integrative Medicine in New York City and author of *The Ageless Woman*. Here are ways to increase your progesterone levels.

Be sure you're getting enough B₆. Since one cause of low progesterone is a vitamin B_6 deficiency, consume foods high in this B vitamin, such as blackstrap molasses, soybeans, and desiccated liver. Also, make sure your supplements contain at least 250 milligrams of B_6, says Dr. Kamhi.

Increase your magnesium intake. Since low magnesium levels are associated with low progesterone, increase your intake of foods high in magnesium, including dark green leafy vegetables and almonds, says Dr. Kamhi. Plus, take 1,000 milligrams a day of magnesium in the form of magnesium glycinate, which is highly absorbable. This will also help with elevated prolactin levels that often accompany low progesterone, Dr. Kamhi says.

Get a prescription for natural progesterone. If you are over 35 or are taking an ovulation-inducing drug such as clomiphene citrate (Clomid), be certain to ask your doctor for a prescription for natural progesterone, such as Crinone or Prometrium, since you will need more to maintain a pregnancy—even if you didn't start out with abnormal levels, stresses Dr. Metzger.

Consider natural progesterone cream. If you aren't taking a prescription medication for progesterone, you might purchase natural progesterone cream over the counter at the health food store, says Dr. Kamhi. Apply ¼ teaspoon to fatty areas of the skin such as the breasts, stomach, and thighs (apply to alternate places with each application). "But more is not better," she cautions. Higher dosages can have a contraceptive effect because the progesterone is converted to estrogen.

Modifying Estrogen

High estrogen levels impair fertility by aggravating endometriosis, fibroids, cysts, and PCOS, in addition to causing other "female problems" like PMS and menopause symptoms. And since hormones work in concert, increased estrogen often means decreased testosterone and progesterone, along with an increase of the antiprogesterone hormone prolactin. This lopsided house of hormone cards is recognized by natural health practitioners as "estrogen dominance." The detoxification protocol described above is the first step toward restoring natural order. In addition, working to bring progesterone levels up should tame unwieldy estrogen. Here's more.

Make your next meal organic. Experts concur that the most important self-care measure to regulate estrogen is to reduce your exposure to "xeno-estrogens" in the environment. Xenoestrogens are aggressive and often carcinogenic molecules that fit into the body's estrogen-receptor sites. They are by-products of the chemical, plastics, and agricultural industry. One way we take them directly into our bodies is by consuming food that contains pesticide residues and hormone-treated animal products. (Also known as endocrine disruptors, xenoestrogens were detailed in chapter 9.) The overarching message for healthy estrogen levels is to make every effort to eat organic food—especially when it comes to meat and dairy products that would otherwise contain synthetic hormones.

Ease stress with relaxation breaks. When you are under chronic stress, your body will convert progesterone into other adrenal hormones, leaving estrogen even more dominant, says Dr. Kamhi. Take relaxation breaks throughout the day—and see chapters 6, 7, and 18 for advice on assessing and managing stress.

Assisting Thyroid

It's not hard to detect low thyroid function that may be too "subclinical" for your doctor to diagnose and treat with medication, says Dr. Kamhi. A dead giveaway is more than a handful of symptoms like sensitivity to cold temperatures, dry skin or hair, chronic fatigue, depression, joint pain, decreased concentration and memory sharpness, irregular menstrual cycles, and low libido. You can also measure how well your thyroid is performing with the help of a basal thermometer (make sure it's glass) by taking your temperature every morning for a month. Before getting out of bed each morning, place the thermometer in your armpit for 10 minutes, then record your temperature. After a month, determine your average temperature. If it's below 97.8 degrees Fahrenheit, you probably have a sluggish thyroid, says Dr. Kamhi. Here are some ways to enhance your thyroid.

Incorporate kelp, seaweed, and other sea vegetables into your diet. They are excellent sources of the iodine that's needed to support a healthy thyroid gland. (Don't take iodine *supplements*, however, because too much can impair the thyroid.) A great food source is California roll (all vegetable) sushi.

Have your iron status checked. Your body must have iron on hand to be able to incorporate iodine into molecules of thyroxine, the main thyroid hormone. (Iodine activates thyroxine.) Make sure any blood tests you have done include a serum ferritin test, which can detect depleted iron stores before you actually become anemic.

Practice some poses. Practicing yoga on a regular basis nourishes the thyroid and helps compensate for the sluggish metabolism that accompanies an underfunctioning thyroid. Two poses that are especially thyroid-stimulating are the Modified Shoulder Stand and the Fish.

Try natural stimulation. A warm castor oil pack placed over the front of the neck, where the thyroid gland is located, can gently stimulate the gland enough to give most women better thyroid levels by 3 months, says Dr. Kamhi. Soak a piece of flannel in castor oil and place it on your neck under a layer of plastic and a warm water bottle wrapped in a towel. Do this for 45 minutes, three times a week. If you don't have time for the pack, try rubbing your palms vigorously together and then placing them over your neck whenever you think of it, recommends Effie Poy Yew Chow, Ph.D., president of East West Academy of Healing Arts in San Francisco, a qigong Grand Master, and coauthor of *Miracle Healing from China—Qigong*.

Consider desiccated thyroid supplements. Naturopaths and integrative physicians are likely to prescribe low doses of desiccated thyroid to support an underfunctioning thyroid. Check with your doctor to see if this option would be beneficial to you.

THE MODIFIED SHOULDER STAND

Lie on your back with your legs bent and your forearms turned out and extended toward your waist with your palms up. Pressing your shoulders down and drawing your shoulder blades toward your waist, bring your palms into your lower back to support it as you gently roll farther back onto your shoulders. Letting your knees come to your forehead, press your elbows into the floor so that no weight is on your neck or cervical spine. If you feel steady, slightly straighten your legs and gaze up at the ceiling for several breaths. Over time, you may "unmodify" the pose so that your legs are vertical. To return your hips to the ground, slowly roll down vertebra by vertebra. Avoid this pose if you have a disk problem, a detached retina, high blood pressure, or are menstruating.

THE FISH

Lying flat on your back, place your hands palms down under your buttocks. Push your forearms and elbows into the ground so that you raise your torso and upper spine with your hips remaining on the ground. Look back behind you until the top of your head touches the ground. Continuing to arch your back and taking the weight into your forearms and elbows, release your hands from under your buttocks and place them palms down beside your hips. Take several calm breaths in this posture. To come out of it, tuck your palms back under your buttocks, use your elbows to lift your head off the ground while you tuck in your chin, and gently release your back into the floor.

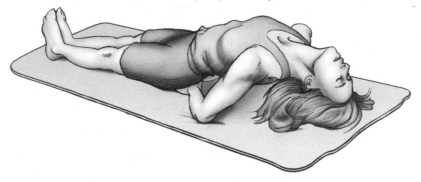

WHAT WORKED FOR US
A LOW-CARB DIET GOT HER HORMONES BACK ON TRACK

Lahle Heninger struggled with a lifelong weight problem, in addition to embarrassing symptoms like acne, baldness, and facial hair. She never menstruated. When she was 27, an endocrinologist told her that her difficulties were caused by a condition called polycystic ovary syndrome (PCOS), which led to a disruption of reproductive hormones, especially an excess of testosterone.

"It was a relief to have an explanation for the symptoms," Lahle remarks. But the treatment at the time was taking birth control pills, and Lahle wanted to start a family. She tried to control her condition with the weight loss strategies and exercises recommended by the endocrinologists she consulted. But on every diet plan she tried, Lahle actually gained *more* weight. In fact, she was accused of cheating on her diets. At 285 pounds, she had difficulty climbing steps, let alone enduring an aerobics class. She finally tried fertility medication anyway, to no avail. At last, Lahle concluded that since her endocrine system seemed to defy childbearing, she would adopt.

After adopting her three children, Lahle heard about a new way to manage PCOS from an online support group. She discovered that rather than the low-fat diets so often being recommended for weight loss, people with insulin conditions such as PCOS needed to focus more on low-*carb* eating. When Lahle did that, the pounds started to melt off.

ENDOCRINE OPTIMIZERS FOR MEN

The same hormone messengers responsible for reproduction in women are at work in men. Luteinizing hormone signals the Leydig cells of the testes to produce testosterone, while follicle-stimulating hormone signals the Sertoli cells to produce sperm. And just as estrogen is essential for egg release, it is also needed by men to produce sperm. Of course, men need significantly less estrogen than women and require much higher levels of testosterone.

That said, the same hormone-balancing recommendations given above for women are also beneficial to men. Following are a few additional guidelines that are particularly helpful for potential dads.

She was originally vigilant about eliminating all carbohydrates, including fruit and all grains. "But now, in the maintenance stage, I worry more about avoiding *processed* foods and refined grains and sugars," she says. If she has a little bread or fruit, she eats it with protein to prevent a surge of the insulin that works against her hormones. She eats only whole grains, since their extra fiber generates less insulin than processed grains.

After losing 135 pounds, Lahle made up for all the years of being sedentary and threw herself into classes at a martial arts gym. Today, she is a black belt. She also regularly enjoys biking, weight lifting, and yoga. Once her acne and skin discoloration disappeared, she discovered newfound self-esteem. A high school dropout, she went back to school to become a registered dietitian—and also started her own business doing video animation. Another thing that came together was her menstrual cycle. As a result of the weight loss, low-carb diet, and fitness routine, it normalized without medication.

Things were going so well—with three beautiful adopted children, a new body, and a new lease on life—that the last thing Lahle and her husband were thinking about was pregnancy. Maybe she wasn't trying for a fourth child, but nature's gift of a little girl perfectly rounded out her caboodle of two adopted boys and an adopted girl.

Take 1 to 4 grams of *Panax ginseng*. Ginseng appears to influence the entire hormone feedback system between the hypothalamus and the testicles. Chinese researchers have noted that even small amounts of *Panax ginseng* caused "obvious stimulating effects on sperm motility with statistical significance." Furthermore, an Italian study found that men who took 4 grams of *Panax ginseng* a day for 3 months doubled their sperm count, and men with a varicocele (a varicose vein of the testicle that can impede the development of normal sperm) increased their sperm count *fourfold*. The men also had statistically significant improvements in testosterone levels. Because of its testosterone effects, *Panax* is not generally advised for women, although other forms of ginseng may be okay, depending on their constitution, says Dr. Lewis.

Supplement with free-radical scavengers. "Oxidative damage is present in at least 25 percent, and possibly up to 75 percent, of the abnormal sperm we see in my practice," says Scott J. Roseff, M.D., director of the West Essex Center for Advanced Reproductive Endocrinology in West Orange, New Jersey, and clinical associate professor in the obstetrics and gynecology department at the University of Medicine and Dentistry of New Jersey. To prevent further free-radical damage, it's essential for men with low or abnormal sperm to take antioxidants (see the recommendations in chapter 3) along with other free-radical scavengers called oligomeric proanthocyanidins (OPCs), he says. Particularly potent sources include extracts of pine bark, red wine extract, grapeseed extract, and bilberry.

Dr. Roseff studied the effect of a formulation of OPCs and other antioxidants called Pycnogenol on subfertile men with marked sperm problems. "After 90 days, the percentage of healthy sperm increased 99 percent, while the number of deformed sperm decreased significantly," he says. "I now prescribe Pycnogenol to all infertile men in my practice." He recommends 200 milligrams a day, along with 30 to 60 milligrams of zinc. You can purchase Pycnogenol over the counter at most health food and drug stores.

Drink almond milk. Nuts, seeds, and legumes contain plant chemicals called phytosterols, which are known to promote testosterone production, says Dr. Lewis. Nuts also contain magnesium, which balances levels of the hormone prolactin, which can compete with testosterone, Dr. Kamhi notes. Great sources of phytosterols and magnesium are almond milk and almond-milk cheese (found at health food stores). Substitute almond milk for cow's milk and you also help prevent the potential estrogenic effects of nonorganic dairy products treated with recombinant bovine growth hormone (rbGH).

17

Integrative Help
for Compromised Organs

To our understanding of the reproductive organs, miniature surgical microscopes, ultrasounds, and internal x-rays have been the equivalent of landing on the moon. The once-inaccessible galaxy in and around the uterus can now be explored, documented, and marveled at. Our probes can scan each tentacle of the fimbria waiting outside the ovaries to whisk up an egg. We can follow the twists and turns of the tubing traveled by sperm and egg as they are waved toward their destiny by microscopic hairs. We have illuminated the pink, spongy landscape of the uterus that waxes and wanes each month in sync with an orbit of hormones. We can also get a clear picture of how any past infection, illness, or injury has left its mark on our reproductive organs. The picture isn't always pretty, but the same space-age technology that allows problems to be detected also allows imperfections to be repaired—or bypassed. Miraculously, scientific advances actually make it possible to remove from the picture one of these three main reproductive organs—ovaries, fallopian tubes, or uterus—and still produce offspring.

A woman with irreparably blocked fallopian tubes can have her eggs fertilized outside her body and placed directly in her womb so that nature can take over from there. A woman whose uterus was removed because of cancer can now have her eggs retrieved, fertilized with her partner's sperm, and grown in another woman's womb. And a woman with no eggs may have donor eggs placed in her own fallopian tubes to meet with her husband's sperm and hopefully grow a baby.

It's good to know that we can fall back on these assisted reproduction technologies when major imperfections are discovered through our amazing imaging techniques. But just because these technologies are available doesn't mean we have to go to the proverbial moon for help if the answer is right at home.

"A lot of doctors will push technologies like in vitro fertilization [IVF]. After all, IVF is very lucrative. Plus a lot of the doctors who do IVF don't feel comfortable doing pelvic microsurgeries that could correct an underlying problem and allow a woman to conceive on her own," comments reproductive endocrinologist and gynecologic surgeon Deborah Metzger, M.D., Ph.D., medical director of Helena Women's Health in San Jose, California, and medical advisor to this book.

"Rather than assuming you need major medical intervention, ask what can be done first to empower the organs you have to work with—despite their imperfections. You may find that some abnormalities aren't really a problem after all," Dr. Metzger says. For example, you don't need both fallopian tubes to be open, or both ovaries to be functioning, to conceive—it just may take longer with only one. And even if you are told you have fibroids or polyps growing in your uterus, don't assume they are a major threat to your fertility, because the great majority of them are benign.

Integrative medicine practitioners can help you to increase your overall vitality, which may improve the function of your reproductive organs enough to get you pregnant without any space-age assistance. When surgery is the intervention of choice, integrative medicine couples it with nutrients, herbs, and other gentle techniques that can create a more favorable outcome. And when assisted reproduction technologies are necessary, integrative medicine offers techniques that can prime the organs for better success rates.

WHEN SURGERY IS AN OPTION

"For men, the varicocele is the most treatable cause of male infertility, and of all the treatment options, surgery offers the highest success rates," says Philip Werthman, M.D., a urologist specializing in male infertility and microsurgery who is the director of the Center for Male Reproductive Medicine and chief of urology at Center City Hospital, both in Los Angeles. A varicocele is an enlargement of the spermatic veins that drain the testicles.

A World Health Organization study noted semen improvement in 70 to 80 percent of men after varicocele surgery and pregnancy rates of up to 60 percent within the first 2 years after successful surgery. Another study found pregnancy rates to be three times higher than among partners of men who didn't opt for the surgery.

Varicocele surgery (called microsurgical inguinal varicocele repair) is performed on an outpatient basis and generally takes 30 to 40 minutes to complete. It is performed through a 1½-inch incision made below the belt line with the assistance of a surgical microscope. The abnormal veins are separated and "tied off" so blood can no longer pool around the testicle, Dr. Werthman explains. "Since a varicocele worsens over time, surgery may be particularly worthwhile for men who plan to father more children in the future," Dr. Werthman says.

In a woman, surgically removing tissue "implants" or lesions caused by endometriosis doubles the chances that a couple will conceive on their own, says Dr. Metzger. In addition, it frees women of debilitating pain they might experience around their periods, as well as other endometriosis symptoms like abdominal discomfort and heavy menses. While removing the lesions doesn't correct the underlying problem, it certainly can allow a couple to gain some time to conceive, since the endometriosis implants don't usually return for several months to several years.

For the small percentage of women with uterine fibroids that might actually interfere with fertility, the two surgical options are uterine artery embolization, which starves the blood vessels supplying the fibroid, or laparoscopic or hysteroscopic myomectomy, in which small fibroids are cauterized or removed. Fibroids recur 30 percent of the time after surgery.

For tubal problems, a surgeon can offer a prognosis of surgical success based on hysterosalpingography (HSG) or falloposcopy. "If the HSG indicates a good prognosis, it's a no-brainer to repair the tubes," says Dr. Metzger.

The chances of a successful outcome are much better if the tube is blocked on one end rather than if both ends are blocked or if a tube is closed all the way through. Pregnancy rates of up to 70 percent can be expected after blockages near the end of the fallopian tubes are repaired. Sometimes this can even be done through a simple catheter procedure rather than surgery. When the blockage is in the middle, a surgeon may be able to remove the part that's blocked and rejoin the rest of the tube. When a tube is so swollen that its diameter is more than four-fifths of an inch or the tubal lining is damaged, however, the prognosis is poor.

Surgery may also be an option if the "male tubes" are obstructed. Pregnancy rates are about 20 to 50 percent after epididymis repair and 50 to 60 percent after vasovasostomy (repair of the vas).

Several congenital abnormalities can be reversed for men and women. Hypospadias (in which a boy is born with the opening of the urethra located under the head or shaft of the penis rather than at the tip) can be repaired easily with surgery. Also very operable is a condition in which a woman's uterus is divided by a thick, fibrous wall called a septum. "Although there's a chance that a woman with a divided uterus can carry a pregnancy, she does have an increased risk of miscarriage. After one or more miscarriages, she's usually advised to look into having the septum removed," says Dr. Metzger.

Of course, surgery is not without its risks. After a couple attempts conception through surgically repaired fallopian tubes, there is an increased chance (around 15 percent) that pregnancies will be ectopic (the egg gets stuck and implants in the tube rather than the ovary). An ectopic pregnancy has to be removed and, if undiagnosed, puts the woman in danger of severe blood loss. In addition, cutting into the organs can create inflammation, scarring, and adhesions—ironically, even if the surgery is performed to do away with these effects because they decrease fertility. Adhesions are found in about 75 percent of women who have had pelvic surgery.

"To reduce your risk of adhesions, ask your surgeon to use an antiadhesion product during the procedure," advises Dr. Metzger. In addition, the integrative medicine advice found in the rest of this chapter combines beautifully with surgery to make your interventions more permanent and effective.

REDUCE ADHESIONS AND TISSUE DAMAGE

The body will lay down bridges of fibrous tissue, also known as collagen cross links, to repair damage from surgery, infection, or trauma. If the inflammation or damage is more serious, the "bridges" will be bigger and are known as adhesions. Wider, thicker bridges are called scars.

People have adhesions all over their bodies. But the reproductive organs are so delicate that they are especially vulnerable to them. Both the fallopian tubes and spermatic tubes are no wider in diameter than a hair. Inflammation or bits of tissue can easily cement them together or get in the way of a sperm or egg's passage. Tougher scar-like surfaces inside the uterus can make it more difficult for an embryo to comfortably sink in and grow. Whether you are preparing for surgery or are concerned about past damage, the following techniques can help heal and nourish the tissues of the reproductive organs.

Apply healing oils. "The herb St. John's wort is so popular for depression that we forget about its other uses. But it's an excellent connective tissue tonic. I recommend using the oil topically over the pelvic organs to reduce adhesions," says Jill E. Stansbury, N.D., a naturopathic physician specializing in reproductive health in Battle Ground, Washington, and chair of the botanical medicine department at the National College of Naturopathic Medicine in Portland, Oregon.

For optimal effect, combine 1 tablespoon of St. John's wort oil with 1 tablespoon of vitamin E oil. If you've just had surgery, put the mixture on a piece of clean fabric and then lay the fabric gently over the top of the

COMMON STRUCTURAL PROBLEMS

There are a number of structural problems in both women and men that could decrease a couple's chances of getting pregnant. Fortunately, most of these can be corrected with surgery or medication. Here are the most common female structural problems.

Congenital abnormalities. Malformations of a woman's reproductive system that occurred while she was still in the womb. Rare abnormalities include having an extra cervical canal, or being born without fallopian tubes or ovaries. More common abnormalities include having a T-shaped uterus that does not leave as much room for a fetus, or a uterus that is divided by a fibrous or muscular wall.

Cystic ovaries. Fluid-filled egg-containing sacs on the ovaries result in abnormal ovulation and can be caused by polycystic ovary syndrome, insulin resistance, or varicose veins of the ovary.

Endometriosis. A disease that results when small pieces of the lining of the uterus (endometrium) implant on tissues and organs of the pelvis. Symptoms can include pelvic pain, pain with intercourse, or infertility. Endometriosis affects more than 5 million U.S. women, 30 to 40 percent of whom are infertile.

Fibroids. Fibroids are benign growths of smooth-muscle tissue, usually between the size of a pea and a tennis ball. Twenty to 30 percent of all women have fibroids, and there is a genetic predisposition. A woman could have one or a cluster of fibroids growing inside the uterus (submucus), through the uterine wall (intramural), or outside the uterus (subserous). Fibroids growing in the uterus could behave as physical barriers to implantation of an egg or stimulate miscarriage, although the chances are slim.

Polyps. Similar to fibroids, polyps are benign masses of tissue that grow out from the endometrium. Because they cause a low-grade inflammation in the endometrium, they can act like an IUD in preventing implantation.

Tubal factors. A blockage or infection anywhere along the delicate finger-lined passage comprising the fallopian tubes. Usually problems occur as a result

fresh wound. If you don't have open wounds, vigorously massage the oils over your abdomen. To encourage the oils to penetrate, you can cover your abdomen with a piece of plastic and add low heat from a heating pad or hot water bottle, Dr. Stansbury adds.

of scarring from past illness or surgery, such as pelvic inflammatory disease or appendicitis.

For men, the most common fertility-compromising structural problems are:

Cryptorchidism. A condition in which a boy is born with testicles inside the abdomen rather than outside the body. Unless it is repaired before a boy is 2 years old, sterility is likely, since undescended testicles won't develop their sperm-generating capacity due to the higher temperature within the abdomen.

Erectile dysfunction. Anything that compromises the circulatory or nervous system can prevent erection. This includes diabetes, medication for high blood pressure, alcohol, atherosclerosis (fatty deposits in the arteries), spinal injuries, and a sedentary lifestyle.

Obstruction of the epididymis. The narrow, coiled tubes where the sperm mature could be blocked by scarring from past infection or inflammation from a current infection. A case of childhood mumps or a sexually transmitted disease is the likely culprit. When antibiotics are given for current infections, semen quality and fertility may return after several months, unless the blockage requires surgery.

Obstruction of the vas deferens. The ejaculatory duct that carries sperm from the epididymis to the penis may have been severed for vasectomy, or it could have been damaged during a past pelvic surgery or malformed in the womb.

Retrograde ejaculation. A congenital abnormality or malfunction of the muscles that normally close off the bladder during ejaculation. It causes semen to move backwards into the bladder instead of being ejaculated through the penis. If medication doesn't help, sperm can be retrieved from the urine through various laboratory techniques.

Varicocele. An enlargement of the spermatic veins, which prevents normal drainage of blood from the testicles. Since the blood tends to pool in the testicles, the temperature of the testes is elevated by about 2 degrees, which impairs sperm and testosterone production. Also, oxygen and nutrients required for sperm development may be restricted. Roughly 40 percent of infertile males have varicoceles, which are easily corrected with surgery.

Use pineapple power. Bromelain is an enzyme found in pineapples that has a number of favorable effects on connective tissues. "I give it to people prior to surgery because it is known to prevent excessive clotting, and it can reduce inflammation and adhesions," says Dr. Stansbury. Sometimes the bromelain pills also contain vitamins such as K, E, and C—and that's beneficial, too, Dr. Stansbury says. Since you'd have to drink gallons of pineapple juice for the same effect, she recommends that you buy bromelain in 500-milligram pills and take two of them, up to three times a day. Start taking the bromelain pills 2 to 3 weeks before going into surgery, and continue to take them until 2 to 3 weeks after surgery, Dr. Stansbury recommends.

Take "green foods." Chlorophyll—that green pigment created when plants react to sunlight—is excellent for healing internal membranes, says Ellen Kamhi, Ph.D., R.N., a health educator and practitioner based in

FERTILITY VISIONARIES

Belinda and Larry Wurn and Clear Passage Therapies

With more than 600 doctors across the country referring their patients to them, Belinda Wurn, a physical therapist, and her husband, Larry Wurn, a massage therapist, had a thriving chain of rehabilitation clinics. Yet Belinda was having trouble managing pain and dysfunction of her own that resulted from previous treatment of cervical cancer.

That's when the Wurns went where no physical and massage therapists had gone before. The couple combined their experiences and developed a method to reduce internal scarring and dysfunction deep in the pelvic organs. Not only did it do wonders for Belinda, but it produced a surprising pregnancy in a patient who was diagnosed with two blocked fallopian tubes and was infertile for 7 years.

Word of mouth spread, and the Wurns found themselves treating women who were considered impossible cases by infertility specialists. One patient came in with a bad case of endometriosis, one blocked tube, one removed tube, and 12 years of infertility, despite numerous surgeries. After treatment, she had a full-term pregnancy at the age of 41. Even health care practitioners who themselves had had no success with medical and surgical infertility treatments came to the Wurns and had successful pregnancies.

Realizing they were onto something, the Wurns received international training in the treatment of the pelvic organs. They hired ob–gyn consultants and

Oyster Bay, New York, who is known as The Natural Nurse. She is the author of *Cycles of Life: Herbs and Energy Techniques for the Stages of a Woman's Life.* Another great green food is sun chlorella, a freshwater, single-celled green algae. It's high in protein, contains every essential amino acid, and helps support tissue repair, she says. Dr. Kamhi recommends 2 to 3 tablespoons a day of powdered chlorophyll, chlorella, or any mixed-greens powder that contains these and other green "superfoods" such as barley grass, various vegetables, and kelp. A great way to take it is by scooping it into a morning protein drink, she says.

Balance your hormones. Endometriosis, fibroids, and ovarian cysts are

devoted their practice to developing the patented "WURN technique."

Clear Passage therapists are trained to identify areas that are tight or have adhesions—often as a result of past infections or injuries. "We use our hands to gently free adhesions in the reproductive tract. We also address any other bodily structures that are creating tensions in the pelvis. It feels like a sustained stretch followed by a tremendous release of tension," Larry Wurn describes. "Our goal is to return normal mobility and function to the affected organs and their neighboring structures."

The success rate at Clear Passage Therapies has been documented by gynecological researchers at 70 percent. Although the WURN technique can be helpful to prepare the uterus for implantation in an assisted reproduction procedure, the success rates are equally high when the technique is performed as a sole treatment.

"Our goal is lasting rehabilitation—that's why several of our patients have gone on to have two or more children after completing their treatment—which you can't say about IVF [in vitro fertilization] or IUI [intrauterine insemination]," Larry Wurn comments.

Contact information: Clear Passage Therapies is located in Gainesville, Florida, but the Wurns also provide 1- or 2-week treatment packages for out-of-town patients. For more information, call (866) BABYHERE or go to www.clearpassage.com.

usually stimulated by estrogen. To prevent these conditions from worsening—or returning after surgery—it's essential to take steps to avoid excess estrogen. It's also important to make sure that your thyroid, adrenal, and insulin levels are balanced as well. Chapter 16 offers detoxification and lifestyle choices that can make a difference. In the case of excess estrogen, your doctor may prescribe birth control pills for their hormone-regulating effects, just up until you are ready to conceive.

INCREASE HEALING CIRCULATION TO YOUR ORGANS

Traditional Chinese Medicine views infertility as one of seven different patterns of imbalance. Encompassing all the Western infertility diagnoses like endometriosis and ovulatory dysfunction, these patterns are described in words like "damp heat," "flem obstruction," "liver qi stagnation," and "blood stasis." "As different as these seven patterns are, they all involve some form of blockage," explains Effie Poy Yew Chow, M.P.H., Ph.D., president of East West Academy of Healing Arts in San Francisco, a qigong Grand Master, and coauthor of *Miracle Healing from China—Qigong*.

Blockages are two-dimensional in Chinese medicine. One type of blockage is a physical obstruction of blood and lymph as they move through the pathways of arteries and veins. The other type is the energetic obstruction of "qi" (the life force) as it moves through pathways called meridians.

"Think about it: If you were poor, would you go to a poor man or a rich man to borrow money? If you have a problem with infertility, you're already a poor man in terms of the reproductive organs. So you have to move your energy and vitality from the rest of the body to the deficient area," explains Dr. Chow.

In Western medicine, we talk about moving white blood cells and nutrients and oxygen instead of qi, but the concept is similar, says Dr. Stansbury. Endometriosis, for instance, causes pain and dysfunction when blood pools up and increases pressure in the blood vessels.

An active lifestyle and regular fitness routine are integral for good circulation. Here are some additional recommendations from both Eastern and Western medicine.

Try hydrotherapy. Hydrotherapy is the use of hot and cold water, traditionally prescribed by naturopathic doctors, to foster healing of all kinds. Dr. Stansbury's hydrotherapy protocol increases circulation to the reproductive organs and is particularly beneficial for relieving endometriosis and varicoceles. Prepare to immerse yourself from the waist down (or at least immerse your pelvic organs) in a basin or tub, she says. You first sit in water as hot as you can stand it for 5 to 10 minutes, then quickly switch to a 30-second soak in cold water. Do this daily for several weeks, Dr. Stansbury advises.

Note: Although men and women are not usually advised to sit in long, hot baths when they are trying to conceive, Dr. Stansbury's regimen is not done for months on end or for long periods of time. Ideally, it will be done for the purposes of getting congestion under control in the *pre*conception period. In the unlikely event that sperm are affected by the heat, they should return to their former condition—or much better—within 3 to 4 months of finishing hydrotherapy.

Get acupuncture. "Acupuncture is the ultimate therapy for improving the flow of blood to finite arteries of the reproductive organs," says Randine Lewis, L.Ac., Ph.D., an oriental medicine doctor with special training in infertility who is director of the Eastern Harmony Acupuncture and Herbal Clinic in Houston. "Not only is acupuncture highly therapeutic for people with compromised organs, but I recommend it for *all* women later in their reproductive years who want to improve their chances of conception," says Dr. Lewis. "Women who are in their early to mid-forties will have about a fifth of the blood supply to the organs as younger women. Acupuncture can actually turn back the clock for their ovaries and uterus," she explains. Dr. Lewis's infertility patients achieve a 75 to 80 percent success rate.

And for women who end up needing IVF, one study showed that those who received two acupuncture sessions (one immediately before and one right after the procedure) had a significantly higher rate of successful implantation (42.5 percent) than women who did not receive acupuncture (26.3 percent). The acupuncture points used were specifically chosen to help relax the uterus and provide sedation, since research shows that uterine contractions when the catheter is transferred through the cervix are associated with poor implantation outcomes.

Take L-arginine and Co-Q$_{10}$ supplements. "L-arginine is an amino acid that actually improves bloodflow to the pelvic organs. Chinese medicine considers it a reproductive tonic," says Dr. Lewis. In fact, a 1999 study documented increased ovarian response, endometrial receptivity, and pregnancy rates in IVF patients who took daily supplements of L-arginine. It has been found to increase sperm count and sperm motility.

Similarly, the enzyme called Co-Q$_{10}$ helps optimize the mitochondria, the powerhouses of the cell. Since Co-Q$_{10}$ supports overall cellular health, it's likely to benefit tissues of the ovaries and uterus, says Dr. Lewis. If your daily multivitamin doesn't already contain L-arginine and Co-Q$_{10}$, they are worth supplementing. (Take the dosage recommended on the product label.)

Give yourself a femoral massage. A femoral massage will send a rush of blood (including healing white cells) to the pelvic organs, says Dr. Lewis. To find the place, lie down on your back with your knees bent and feel around in the crease in your groin (where most underwear hits). You should feel a pulsing slightly outside of the midpoint of that crease, toward the hip bone. Massage this place for 30 seconds on each side, three times a day, she says. The femoral massage is not advised for people with high blood pressure, glaucoma, or varicoceles.

Consume less dairy, more water. Although Western medicine doesn't pay much attention to phlegm (mucus) unless you have a cold, Eastern medicine recognizes phlegm as one of the underlying causes of infertility. "Phlegm tends to accumulate in the lower parts of the body, obstructing the free flow of qi and blood," says Wei Liu, M.P.H., T.C.M.D., a doctor of Chinese medicine; clinical professor at the American Academy of Acupuncture and Oriental Medicine in Roseville, Minnesota; and author of *Chinese Medicine for Infertility*. You can reduce phlegm by cutting way back on dairy products and making sure you're drinking no less than eight 8-ounce glasses of water a day. Try to incorporate the Daikon radish into your diet, too, Dr. Liu adds. In addition to being known as a phlegm-cleansing food, it is also very hydrating.

ALIGN YOUR ANATOMY

Physical therapists, massage therapists, qigong teachers, and other practitioners who focus on body alignment and muscular imbalances see a common denominator in the infertile clients they work with: a history of back, hip, and neck discomfort. Infertile couples are commonly stressed-out couples, and back pain and other structural problems are often the end result of chronic stress, notes Dr. Metzger.

"More specifically, we find that women with infertility tend to have tightness in their hips and back because their cervix is pulled to one side— maybe from a fall off a horse or a gymnastic accident years ago. We also see a lot of cases where the spine or hips are thrown out of line, which can contribute to poor sperm quality, or adhesions, or a spastic uterus," says Larry Wurn, L.M.T., a licensed massage therapist and codirector of the physical therapy–based infertility program Clear Passage Therapies in Gainesville, Florida.

"Even the infertility treatment itself can create or exacerbate structural problems," explains Nataly Pluta, P.T., A.Y.T., a physical therapist and yoga therapist who runs Pluta Movement Therapeutics in Del Mar, California. "As a woman goes through the infertility workups and treatments, she is all too often put into stirrups for extended periods of time and under stressful circumstances. This alone can cause muscle tightness in the hip area, which can compress the reproductive organs," she explains.

"From an Eastern medicine perspective, a tight back is a problem because that's where the kidneys are—the organs that govern sexual energy," says Dr. Chow. "And the neck controls all the energy channels going up and down the body. If you just loosen the neck, it will already begin to improve circulation to the pelvic organs. Posture, and the way a person breathes, are responsible for a lot of structural tension and imbalance, even if a person never experienced a major injury," Dr. Chow adds.

"Not only will infertility patients benefit by receiving bodywork to correct underlying imbalances, but they should take up a regular practice like yoga or tai chi to increase self-awareness of their posture and breath," says Pluta. Here are some techniques from those therapeutic, Eastern disciplines.

Breathe like a baby. "Think of the way a baby breathes from the moment it is born," says Dr. Chow. "It doesn't move its shoulders up and down; it moves its belly in and out. And when a baby hears a loud noise, it doesn't draw its shoulders in—it flails its arms out and releases that pent-up energy and then relaxes. If we really watch them, they can teach us a lot." Make mental notes throughout the day to breathe with your diaphragm (where the rib cage ends, above the navel) so the air moves your belly and expands your ribs like an accordion, rather than using your upper body. Stretch your arms in all directions and then let your shoulders rest in a loosely rolled back, not forward, position—even when you are under duress.

Add imagery. "The *baiwei* is the point at the top of your head known in Chinese medicine as Conception Vessel #20. Imagine a silver thread through the baiwei," says Dr. Chow. "Let it come out from there, reaching up to heaven and stretching your spine so that no vertebrae [are] compressing onto one another. Again, remember to breathe with your diaphragm and relax your shoulders."

Rotate your hips. First, stand up and rub your palms vigorously together, making sure the center points of your palms make contact, recommends Dr. Chow. This intensifies circulation and brings a lot of blood to the pelvic organs, she says. When your hands are hot, place them over your kidneys, on your lower back. Now, keeping your upper body still, move your hips like you're doing a slow hula dance, 10 times on each side. Take one breath for each rotation, and make your circles as big and as slow as possible. "This massages all your internal organs and wakes up their energy. Not only does it reduce back pain, but we've eliminated fibroids using the hip rotation." she comments.

Release your spine and hips. The yoga pose known as the Pigeon stretches, strengthens, and tones the spinal column and hip joints and groin muscles. It is part of a series of poses recommended for infertility by the American

THE PIGEON

The Pigeon pose stretches the spine, hips, and groin. From a kneeling position, slide your left leg straight back and sit on your right heel. Bend forward and rest your chest on your right thigh, as you allow your hips to open a little more so your right heel can inch closer to your left hip. Place your hands palms down near your shoulders or, for an additional stretch, reach your arms straight out in front of you.

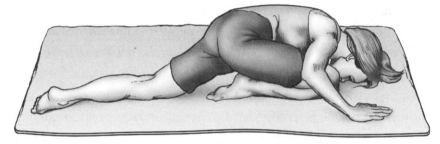

After five full breaths, keep your legs as they are, but place your hands beside your bent knee. Use your hands to support your upper body as you raise it as far as you can into a gentle arch. (Rising up on your fingertips will help you extend the stretch.) Look up, and take five breaths. To come out of the posture, curl your toes under and push back into a kneeling position. Repeat all movements on the other side.

Yoga Association. Ideally, the Pigeon pose should be part of a daily 30- to 90-minute yoga practice led by an experienced teacher, says Pluta. Infertility patients who study yoga as part of Pluta's Seat of the Soul program in Del Mar, California, have achieved over 70 percent success with natural or IVF pregnancies. Seat of the Soul is endorsed by the International Association of Yoga Therapists and RESOLVE: The National Infertility Association.

CALM AND TONE YOUR UTERUS

If the uterus goes into spasm after ovulation, it can prevent the egg from implanting and growing. Other times, the embryo implants but a hyperexcitable uterine muscle aborts it. "We don't know exactly why this happens, but it seems that for some people, their nerve endings are hyperexcitable in the way some people have a tendency to get hives or allergies," says Dr. Stansbury. "Any mild inflammation could lead to the irritated nerve endings."

"These problems could also be caused by lack of abdominal muscle tone. It's similar to the way a person who works out may get a little muscle soreness after a day of raking leaves, while a sedentary person has all-out muscle spasms. Someone who is obese or has chronic constipation might not hold things in place as well as someone with better tone. The uterus can also be stretched out after a number of pregnancies," Dr. Stansbury adds.

Fortunately, midwives and herbalists have thousands of years of experience at toning the uterus with botanical medicine. Here are some of the tried-and-true remedies.

Combine crampbark with blue cohosh. "Crampbark is my ace in the hole for uterine irritability or a hyperexcitable uterine muscle that leads to chronic miscarriage," says Dr. Stansbury. "It combines well with blue cohosh, another classic uterine tonic and female herb." Dr. Stansbury's typical protocol is to combine equal amounts of the liquid tinctures of crampbark and blue cohosh and take 1 teaspoon two to three times a day. It can be taken for 2 to 3 months, she says.

Be sure to supplement fatty acids. Essential fatty acids (EFAs) are "good" fats needed for the membranes of your brain cells as well as the production of cervical mucus. "They also help you maintain healthy uterine membranes so you can get an egg to stick. Plus, your body uses up a tremendous amount of EFAs to maintain a pregnancy, so it's important to be well-supplied," says Jan Hanson, L.Ac., M.S., a nutrition-based integrative medicine practitioner in San Rafael, California, and the coauthor of *Mother Nurture*. "As essential as they are, fatty acids are probably the single largest deficiency in the United States. Almost everyone is deficient if they aren't supplementing," she says. Hanson advises taking 1,000 milligrams a day of a purified fish oil supplement. If you are a vegetarian, the next best thing is flax oil.

Drink raspberry tea. Red raspberry is like yoga for the uterus—this herb simultaneously firms and relaxes the pelvic muscles and ligaments. It also eases childbirth and can reduce hemorrhage, says Dr. Kamhi. Consuming it regularly is a good habit to get into when you're trying to conceive because it's helpful throughout your pregnancy. Raspberry leaf is loaded with nutrients such as calcium and iron, and it enriches colostrum, the immune-stimulating first milk of nursing mothers. For optimum effect, steep 1 teaspoon of loose tea from the leaves of red raspberry per cup of water. The tea is soothing and has a mild flavor, Dr. Kamhi says.

18

The Mind–Body Approach for Unexplained and Secondary Infertility

Seeking out the 21st century's most cutting-edge technologies to solve their fertility problems, 200 infertility patients signed up for in vitro fertilization (IVF) or IVF and intracytoplasmic sperm injection (ICSI) at a Korean hospital. For four cycles, they all took the same fertility medications. Each woman also had three eggs fertilized with her partner's sperm and placed in her uterus. What they didn't know is that half of them also received one of humankind's most ancient and mysterious interventions: They were being prayed for by people on the other side of the world.

The IVF patients who weren't being prayed for averaged a typical pregnancy rate for the procedure: 26 percent. Those who were randomly selected for prayer intervention had nearly *double* the success, with 50 percent of them becoming pregnant! The Columbia University researchers who organized and documented the study are positive that it was airtight. Volunteers in the United States, Canada, and Australia did not know the Korean patients they prayed for. Neither the patients nor their doctors knew about the intervention. The randomized, double-blind study setup ruled out any placebo effect, making the stunning success of prayer difficult for the researchers to explain.

"I'm impressed, but not at all surprised, by the results of the prayer study. After treating infertile couples for more than 20 years, I've found that it's not unusual when the reason for not conceiving—or the solution—is on a more spiritual and psychological level than what hard science can explain," comments Michael R. Mantell, Ph.D., assistant clinical professor in the department of psychiatry at the University of California, San Diego Medical School. Dr. Mantell is also a clinical psychologist at Grossmont Medical Center in La Mesa, California, who specializes in the care and treatment of couples struggling with infertility.

"Unexplained infertility" is the medical diagnosis given after a complete infertility workup reveals no concrete problems with the organs or hormones that control reproduction, yet the couple doesn't conceive after a year or more of trying. Between 10 and 15 percent of infertility patients are given this label. Approximately half of miscarriages are also labeled "unexplained" because no genetic or physical abnormalities are found.

Another subgroup of people test positive for physical problems, like endometriosis, or hormonal problems, like low progesterone. Yet even after these abnormalities are corrected, their infertility continues. Other couples are diagnosed with "secondary infertility" after having a successful pregnancy in the past but difficulty conceiving when they try again. Rarely, women develop a physical problem as a result of their last pregnancy, like pelvic inflammatory disease. More commonly, secondary infertility doesn't have a medically explainable cause.

Unexplained infertility is sometimes treated with the same medications and assisted reproduction procedures used for concrete cases of infertility, with modest success. But infertility specialists grapple with sinking so much time and money into an unclear condition. In fact, the American Society for Reproductive Medicine suspects that those with unexplained infertility who do conceive while getting conventional medical treatment for infertility would have eventually conceived on their own. Meanwhile, the rest of couples with unexplained infertility who don't respond to medical intervention have used up all the conventional options.

Like prayer, modalities that work through the spirit or the mind are showing anecdotal and documented successes for even the trickiest cases of infertility. These modalities include hypnosis, cognitive–behavioral therapy, biofeedback, healing touch, visualization, affirmation, support groups, and other forms of psychotherapy, self-help, and mind–body therapy. Some mind–body visionaries go so far as to say that the psycho-spiritual element is *the* missing link to medically unexplained infertility.

Consider the case of a group of secondary infertility patients who sought out psychological intervention. After 18 months, researchers documented a 60 percent pregnancy rate, compared to the meager 10 percent pregnancy rate of the secondary infertility patients who didn't seek psychological intervention. Along the same lines, Harvard Medical School researchers found that infertile couples who participated in a support group or underwent 10 weeks of cognitive–behavioral therapy had pregnancy rates higher than 50 percent, in contrast to rates of only 20 percent among infertile couples who used conventional medicine alone.

Practitioners can't always pinpoint how mind–body therapies work, but a growing body of research is beginning to map out the mind's role in multiple systems that govern reproduction, including the immune system, the nervous system, and the hormone pathways between the brain and the ovaries (or testes).

THE PSYCHOSOMATIC SIDE OF INFERTILITY

"An innate, evolutionary survival mechanism is often at play when a couple is having trouble conceiving," says clinical psychologist Elizabeth Muir, Ph.D., a London-based specialist in the area of unexplained infertility who directs the Fertility Enhancement Therapy Group. "A female animal is predisposed to turn off her reproductive functions when any kind of a threat to her or her future offspring's survival is perceived," she explains.

Think of yourself as a mama bear, getting ready for mating season. Like any sexually mature animal, you will seek out everything you need for short- and long-term security. You'll need an acceptable level of health, a suitable (and where necessary, also supportive) mate, a territory appropriate to sustain offspring, and a threat-free nesting site (or bear den).

"The failure to maintain all of these factors to a satisfactory level will interfere with the procreative process," Dr. Muir explains. That's why it's essential to examine your environment, lifestyle, and relationships to determine if they are nurturing—or possibly sending your animal brain a message that it's "unsafe" to reproduce.

Whereas simpler animals have only genetically motivated considerations to cope with, humans have an added factor: Our subconscious mind stores all the experiences of our lives going back to the womb. A woman may consciously want a baby, but her subconscious may be at work in a protective way to stop her from reproducing, Dr. Muir says. A powerful factor is unresolved trauma from past abuse.

When Brown University researchers polled 732 women of childbearing age, those who experienced physical or sexual violence in their childhood or teen years had abnormally low estrogen levels and abnormally elevated levels of follicle-stimulating hormones in their thirties and forties, which disrupted the regulation of their ovaries. The abused women were more likely to experience premature menopause than other women.

Conscious thoughts can also trigger inappropriate arousal of our brain's fertility-protective mechanisms, says Dr. Muir. She calls these the "what-if" influences. Negative messages can be related to relationship issues ("What if he leaves me?"), pregnancy issues ("What if my baby is disabled?"), childbirth issues ("Everyone says it's painful, I can't bear the pain"), or parenting apprehension ("I'm sure I will not be able to cope"). Unchallenged thought patterns like these will provoke mood changes, anxiety, depression, physical tension, and belief-fulfilling behavior—any of which can compromise fertility, Dr. Muir asserts.

"Psychosomatic factors in no way mean that it's your fault that you're infertile," Dr. Muir stresses. They are genetic impulses stemming from your brain. The beauty of mind–body therapy is that it enables you to create new communications between your mind and your body that support reproduction.

PRACTICE POSITIVE CONDITIONINGS

As with any other infertility diagnosis, the older you are and the more time that passes, the more your chances of conceiving drop. But before you confuse the label of un*explained* infertility with un*resolvable* infertility, note that statistically, 76 percent of couples with unexplained infertility conceive within 2 years, as do many in their third year.

Don't let miscarriage foil your confidence, either. Even after two losses, 60 percent of couples carry their next pregnancy to term, and after three losses, 40 percent of couples still have successful pregnancies. All too often, people latch on to the false belief that they just aren't "meant" to get pregnant, Dr. Muir says. "This problem is particularly prevalent in couples over the age of 35, who, by no coincidence, have the highest rates of unexplained infertility."

Because of the power of the mind on conception, you must consciously work against letting a diagnosis of unexplained infertility become a natural contraceptive. "The belief system is very important, and it plays a crucial role in the success of reproduction," asserts Dr. Muir.

The following advice will put your mind on your side.

Avoid "too-oldisms." If you're older, you're vulnerable to all kinds of negative reinforcement, like talk that your eggs are no good or your time is up. Don't focus too much on your age—the most important factor for successful conception is *not* your age but what is going on in your life and how you react to it. *That* you can control, says Dr. Muir.

Think in the affirmative. Dr. Mantell relates a tale of two infertile couples: One held off buying a crib and stroller, and the other got the nursery ready as if the baby would arrive tomorrow. "Sure enough, the couple who bought the crib got pregnant, and the other couple didn't," he reports.

"I'm not saying to go out and buy baby stuff. But you should be absolutely convinced that you're going to get pregnant," Dr. Mantell clarifies. You have to start thinking and acting like a mother to make positive conditioning work for you. Rid your mind of any doubt by saying *when* I get pregnant, not *if*. "In fact, I discourage the use of the term *unexplained infertility* altogether. Just call it not-yet-explained subfertility," he says.

Create a picture-perfect future. A powerful visualization to help make your dreams come true is offered by Ellen Kamhi, Ph.D., R.N., a health educator and practitioner based in Oyster Bay, New York, who is known as The Natural Nurse. She is the author of *Cycles of Life: Herbs and Energy Techniques for the Stages of a Woman's Life.* Get a large piece of cardboard and cut out pictures from magazines to create a collage, she says. Fill it up with pictures of pregnant women, babies, dads, families, and whatever else conjures the scenes you would like to play out in your own life. Place the completed collage near your bed and gaze at it as you are falling asleep. In your mind's eye, watch a movie where you enter the scenes, Dr. Kamhi instructs. After a week or two of doing this exercise, you may start to have dreams about the family you will have. "In a mystical way, your body may be prompted to bring this vision into reality," she says. We may never know how it works, but "it often does the trick," she assures.

TAKE A LEAP OF FAITH

"You'll have an easier time with infertility after making peace with the concept that there aren't always medical answers," says Dr. Mantell. When couples become consumed with finding something to blame for their infertility, they might start to make up reasons for not conceiving that become self-limiting. In the case of secondary infertility, they might think that if they had been a better parent with their first child, they would be able to have a second one, or they might rationalize that they are being punished for something in their past. "These are irrational or erroneous explanations," Dr. Mantell says. "It's also unproductive to focus a lot of blame on your partner or your doctor," he adds.

Conceiving takes trust in yourself, your mate, your health care team, and the life forces that you believe in. "If you come from a faith tradition, you're fortunate to be able to extend your hopes and fears to a power bigger than you," says Dr. Mantell. "Attending synagogue, going to church, and studying your Bible or holy book can be a great comfort." In the Judeo-Christian tradition, you can read about how Sarah, Rachael,

REPRODUCTIVE IMMUNOLOGY: AN EXPLANATION FOR MISCARRIAGE AND UNEXPLAINED INFERTILITY?

Although doctors used to think that 15 to 20 percent of pregnancies ended in miscarriage, reproductive health organizations such as the American College of Obstetricians and Gynecologists and RESOLVE: The National Infertility Association now recognize that pregnancy loss may be as high as 70 percent. It is estimated that more than half of these losses go undetected because they occur so close to conception (before symptoms or lab tests reveal the pregnancy). Not only do these previously unrecognized miscarriages seem to explain some cases of unexplained infertility, but they may be treatable—thanks to the growing medical field of reproductive immunology. The study of immune system abnormalities that affect pregnancy has been adopted by pioneers in the field of microbiology, immunology, pathology, genetics, endocrinology, infectious diseases, pediatrics, obstetrics, and gynecology.

"Our scientific research and experimental treatments are showing that patients do not necessarily have to accept statements like 'your miscarriage was meant to be,' 'you are just unlucky,' or 'your eggs are too old,'" comments Alan Beer, M.D., director of the reproductive medicine program at Finch University of Health Sciences at Chicago Medical School and one of the forefathers of reproductive immunology.

The two broad categories of reproductive immune abnormalities are *alloimmune* and *autoimmune* responses. With alloimmune problems, an incompatibility between the woman's and the man's contributions to a pregnancy prevents the woman's body from properly recognizing it. For example, a woman's natural killer cells that normally help her fight disease may recognize the embryo as a foreign invader and prevent it from implanting.

Rivka, Hana, and Leah managed their infertility and not feel so alone, he comments. You can also add your name to prayer requests through your worship group, Dr. Mantell relates.

Even if you don't practice a formal religion and aren't comfortable

Autoimmune responses occur when a woman's body blocks her own biological mechanisms that support a pregnancy. Most commonly, she has elevated antiphospholipid antibodies that cause her blood to clot too fast. This disorder can cause a number of adverse effects in a pregnancy, including compromised exchange of nutrients and waste products between mother and fetus. Reproductive immunologists are finding that antiphospholipid antibodies are an underlying cause of recurrent miscarriages and possibly endometriosis, premature ovarian failure, and unexplained infertility as well.

Aspirin and aspirin combined with heparin (a blood thinner) are among the first treatments used to overcome the blood clots and inflammatory reactions characteristic of immunological problems. For more aggressive treatment, the steroid prednisone is prescribed to decrease autoantibody levels, clotting, and inflammation. The last resort is a more invasive (and highly expensive) procedure in which a woman is infused with antibodies from thousands of blood donors, called intravenous immunoglobulin. The introduced antibodies appear to either keep her own antibodies too busy to attack the developing fetus or contain the pregnancy-supporting antibodies that her mate was unable to provide.

"Since the immune system can be depressed by emotional turmoil from the miscarriage itself, or turmoil in one's past, I recommend that any medical intervention is also combined with mind–body therapies," adds Niravi Payne, M.S., a psychotherapist in Sanibel, Florida, specializing in mind–body treatment of infertility and author of *The Whole Person Fertility Program*.

Reproductive immunology is still considered relatively controversial, but even conventional medical societies recommend immune testing if you are 35 or older and have experienced either two miscarriages or two failed attempts at in vitro fertilization (IVF), or if you are under 35 and have had three miscarriages or three failed IVF attempts. For more information, contact the reproductive medicine program at Finch University of Health Sciences, 3333 Green Bay Road, North Chicago, IL 60064, or e-mail info@repro-med.net.

with prayer, you can still put out the mental, psychic energy to the universe that you wish to sustain a pregnancy, says Dr. Kamhi.

Here are some more mystical methods to foster trust and patience as you journey toward parenthood.

Connect with life-giving forces. "The energy field that surrounds us—call it aura, bioelectric energy, chi, or life force—has an innate intelligence. It 'knows' our challenges, stresses, and limits, perhaps better than our ego-based mind," says Dr. Kamhi. "Make it clear to this higher power that you have the time, space, love, and patience needed for parenthood." For some women, this might mean a personal ritual where you burn sage and call out to your grandmothers to hear your intention to continue the family line, she suggests.

Resolve spiritual conflicts. If you had a bad experience in the past that keeps you from experiencing the support of a faith community, you may need to come to terms with those old wounds, says Dr. Mantell. "Try to put it in perspective," he offers. "If you were in a horrible car accident when you were a kid, does that stop you from driving? You probably don't say that all cars are not good. Do you really believe that all religion is bad, and that every minister is a fake, or can you admit that your views are based on only a few experiences?"

Meditate on life and youth. "The *Dan Tien* meditation allows you to literally breathe life into and through your reproductive organs. I used it myself before conceiving my daughter," says Randine Lewis, L.Ac., Ph.D., an oriental medicine doctor with special training in infertility. She directs the Eastern Harmony Acupuncture and Herbal Clinic in Houston.

When you are in a relaxed state, visualize light entering your body through the top of your head with each inhalation. This light is clean and pure and represents the energy of life and youth. Allow this light to pass through the base of your brain. See it enter the pituitary gland, which is located behind the center of your eyebrows. On another inhalation, bring the focus down to the midline of your body, between your breasts, and then down to your abdomen, eventually focusing your breath in the region 2 inches below your navel. This is called the *Dan Tien*, where our life source begins. Let the breath energy pool here for several breaths. Feel light and purity wash over your reproductive organs, and then return the light back the way it came—up the midline of the body and back through the top of your head. Repeat the meditation over and over until the movements become smooth and continuous, instructs Dr. Lewis.

RELEASE EMOTIONAL BAGGAGE

As important as it is to heal from the past, we are culturally predisposed to bury our wounds very deep down where they are difficult to access. In a philosophy stemming back to the Victorian era, children are often taught that they are to be seen and not heard. The message: Our emotions have to be held in, from the best to the most negative and hurtful. The place they get stored is often the center of the body, where the heart and reproductive organs reside, says Carista Luminare-Rosen, Ph.D., a California-based counselor who specializes in holistic approaches to preconception and is the author of *Parenting Begins before Conception*.

Unresolved guilt about an abortion, grief over a miscarriage, ambivalence, and the humiliation from past abuses are common issues that are stored up, notes Dr. Luminare-Rosen. "On a physical level, emotional blockages stored near the ovaries and uterus can potentially manifest as tight abdominal tissues that impair bloodflow. On an energetic level, emotional blockages can prevent your natural vitality from circulating throughout your reproductive system," she says.

Mind–body techniques, like those that follow, can help us let go of the blockages and heal on the deepest levels.

Uncover hidden ambivalence. "You may be unaware that part of you is saying yes to a pregnancy while part of you is saying no," says Niravi Payne, M.S., a psychotherapist in Sanibel, Florida, specializing in mind–body treatment of infertility and author of *The Whole Person Fertility Program*. Even if you consciously think you want to get pregnant, be honest and try to make a list of reasons for possibly not wanting a child, she says. Write the first thing that comes to your mind. The primary reasons women most often give include fear of losing control of their lives, repeating their parents' mistakes, losing financial independence, experiencing career setbacks, experiencing body changes, and losing closeness with their mates, she says. "Many people mistakenly believe that admitting and discussing their negative feelings about having children will somehow prevent them from becoming pregnant, but my experience with my clients proves quite the opposite. Let these fears come through from your subconscious mind so you can address and release them."

Take an emotional x-ray. "I recommend mentally scanning the abdominal area for images and feelings. When old wounds are located, let that part of the body talk from its point of view to tell you how to let it go," says Dr. Luminare-Rosen. For instance, you might perceive a fiery red ball in your womb that indicates anger. Probe deeper and you might discover the need to forgive your last husband for not wanting children.

"Choose a safe and comfortable environment, like a favorite place in nature, or in your bedroom with soothing music playing," Dr. Luminare-Rosen instructs. "Close your eyes and place your hand on your abdomen. As you slow your breathing, sense the quality of the energy that comes from your womb and any images that emerge. Is it dense, fluid, dark, light, open, closed, a certain color? These feelings and images should offer clues to what kind of attention your reproductive system needs. The action to take next may be getting therapy, writing a letter to a person you have suppressed emotions about, speaking to your partner about inhibitions, or asserting unexpressed needs to your boss, parents, or partner."

Grieve past losses. "If you have ever miscarried, even if it was early on, it is a big deal and needs closure," says Payne. She also encourages women to let go of any despair, guilt, or anger about a past abortion. Healing can be facilitated through a "grief ceremony," she says.

To prepare for a grief ceremony, Payne recommends writing a letter addressed to "my dearly missed child" (or to the child's name if you had one picked out). Explain to the child either why its life was important to you, or why you couldn't support its life at the time. Also tell the child why you feel it is necessary to release it—and maybe add that you would be grateful if its spirit should return to you, she says. Conclude your letter with words that help you feel a sense of closure, such as "Goodbye, I love you, and I have to let you go so your soul can travel on."

Now pick a day to hold a grief ceremony where you will read the letter out loud in the presence of one or two close friends or your partner. It is helpful to use a prop to focus on, such as a bouquet of flowers or a doll.

You may also fly a balloon or paper kite that represents your unborn children, and then release it into the wind, Payne advises.

Heal with hypnotherapy. Hypnosis is a powerful therapeutic tool that enables women to access the relevant issues that might trigger psychosomatic infertility and resolve them, explains Dr. Muir. "Increased sensory perception and heightened control allow a person to use her own resources and skills to deal with her issues of infertility. She'll also experience healthy biochemical changes like the production of endorphins, which are morphine-like substances naturally produced by the body to create a state of comfort," she says. Dr. Muir primarily treats couples with unexplained infertility and reports an average of 60 percent pregnancy rates after hypnotherapy treatment. To locate a hypnotherapist in the United States, contact the American Board of Hypnotherapy's referral service in Santa Ana, California, at (800) 872-9996.

SPECIAL SELF-CARE FOR INFERTILE MOMS

"Having your first child was a major life change that probably altered your sense of security and well-being in countless ways," says Payne. You may feel more financially vulnerable, your division of labor with your spouse may have changed, and you may feel more emotionally isolated than you did before your first child. "In my experience, I find that it is important for a woman to closely examine the events that have affected her psychologically since she gave birth, in order to truly understand what is happening to prevent another pregnancy," says Payne.

Since conceiving your last child, your physical health may have taken as many hits as your psyche. Although most people need 7 to 9 hours of sleep a night, the average mom gets 6 to 6½ hours of sleep nightly, and the quality is worse. And 9 out of 10 mothers don't meet basic nutritional requirements before conceiving their first child. Then, pregnancy and breastfeeding take the best reserves of the nutrients they do have.

"Because of these physical and emotional vulnerabilities, at least 1 out of 10 new mothers goes through a severe degree of depletion 1 to 3 years after a baby is born. For women with preexisting health problems, or women who are having kids at an older age, the figure is probably more like two out of three," says Rick Hanson, Ph.D., a clinical psychologist in northern California who specializes in parental stress and family issues. The depletion Dr. Hanson describes is marked by both physical and emotional exhaustion. After seeing common symptoms among his patients and in his research, he identified it as "depleted mother syndrome" and coauthored a book about resolving it called *Mother Nurture.*

Whether you feel completely depleted or are simply trying to increase your fertility while being a healthy mom, the following advice is for you.

Cultivate community. In modern times, the village it takes to raise a child often looks more like a ghost town, notes Dr. Hanson. Not only do children thrive best in a nurturing community of loving relatives, friendly neighbors, and supportive institutions, but mothers do, too. "The tasks and the cares of parenting are meant to be shared with other mothers and fathers who can lend a hand and lift our spirits," he says. Be proactive about reaching out to other parents, like starting a play group or babysitting co-op, joining a mothers' club, or using the Internet. You're also welcome to join the virtual community of mothers and the people who love them at www.nurturemom.com, says Dr. Hanson.

Savor mothering moments. Moms have so many positive experiences in a day, but many mothers are so task-oriented or self-sacrificing they often don't let themselves slow down and really have that experience. "When you have positive experiences, take that moment of mindfulness to let it sink in deep to your emotional memory so it becomes a part of your soul," says Dr. Hanson. Over time, those positive experiences become great resources for coping with stress.

Maintain your sense of self. Motherhood is a sacred role, but it doesn't have to be your sole identity. It can help take the pressures off motherhood to expand your interests in other areas. You could return to an interest you had before children, such as playing a musical instrument, writing letters to help free political prisoners, or bicycle touring. If you're currently a homemaker, you might want to put efforts into staying up-to-date in your last career. Or take up a new interest.

Master sound sleep. As discussed earlier, loss of sleep is a major reason why many mothers of young children feel so depleted that they can't support another pregnancy. Some suggestions: If you're home with the babies, take naps during the day when they do instead of turning to housework. Also, make sure your kids don't have any health problems, like allergies, that could be waking them up, offers Dr. Hanson. If they do, be sure they get proper medical treatment. In addition, negotiate with your partner to take over more of the overnight parenting.

Improve intimacy. Between sleep deprivation and putting all their focus on children, most new parents simply don't have thriving sexual lives. It may help to alleviate resentment and anxiety to recognize that a temporary disinterest in sex is biological and not a reflection of your affection for one another. Discuss how to stay intimate as a couple if you can't have sex with the same frequency as you did pre-baby.

Examine financial vulnerability. One of the major reasons women struggle with both primary and secondary infertility is their fear that they will no longer be self-sufficient, says Payne. If you grew up seeing an intense frustration over your mother's economic dependence on your father, discuss with your partner how things can be different. However the money comes in, you may have to move to a higher level of trust and understanding that you're both equally entitled to your common resources.

Rearrange your division of labor. Even in households where a husband contributes to the domestic workload, when the mother works outside the home, women work roughly 15 hours longer each week than most men. Add that up, and over a year, that's an entire month of 24-hours-straight extra labor—clearly a negative stressor. You and your mate will need tremendous flexibility as you experiment with adjustments in careers, child care, and lifestyle choices that work best for your family. Have you considered options like telecommuting, self-employment, or a trial of Mr. Mom?

19

Coming to Terms with Infertility

Infertility creates turmoil in almost every aspect of a woman's and a couple's life. No part of life is left unaffected: Trips to the shopping mall, visits with family and friends, introductions to new acquaintances, intimacy and sexuality, childhood memories—even dreams for the future—are all touched when a woman who wants children is unable to conceive or carry a child to term.

Getting through infertility requires some extra effort, just when you have the least energy. But it's important to take care of yourself and your relationship—after all, your goal is to become parents at the end of this marathon. Support groups offer a wealth of strength to many infertile women and couples, and infertility counseling can provide more focused help when making one more decision seems impossible.

As we've discussed throughout this book, there is a wide array of treatment options—including medication, surgery, and integrative medicine strategies—to help couples who are struggling with infertility. Yet at a certain point, you will know that it is time to come to resolution. If you've been undergoing assisted reproduction techniques without luck, you may need to discontinue such heroic steps for emotional, physical, or financial reasons—or all three. If you've been unsuccessful getting pregnant on your own and decide not to pursue medical treatment for religious or other personal reasons, resolution may come sooner. In cases like these, coming to closure after infertility often happens in one of two ways: adopting or remaining child-free. Coming to terms with infertility is a complex process. Fortunately, there are a number of active steps you can take to win back a sense of control and move toward a full and healthy life.

REGAIN CONTROL

Women struggling with infertility share many concerns—but the biggest one may be a loss of control over their bodies and their lives. "There is not a single person going through infertility who feels in control," says Sonia Hieger, C.S.W., an infertility psychologist in Manhasset, New York.

Feeling out of control means that decision-making is difficult or impossible. Lack of control over how people perceive you or how much they know of your personal life can tempt normally social individuals to become hermits. At the extreme, loss of control can lead to scary physical symptoms, adding panic and anxiety to an already stressful time. Experts recommend that women going through infertility actively try to regain control over whatever they can. These tips can help.

Make a timeline. Whether you are undergoing assisted reproduction techniques or taking natural steps to conception, making a clear plan of action offers a real measure of control, says Linda D. Applegarth, Ed.D., director of psychological services at the Center for Reproductive Medicine and Infertility and clinical assistant professor of psychology at New York Presbyterian Hospital–Weill Medical Center of Cornell University in New York City. "There are so few things you can be in control of in this situation," she notes. "I encourage couples to work with their doctors to develop a clear treatment plan, and write it down." Your actual treatment decisions can alter your plans along the way, of course. But there is a certain amount of comfort in having a clear but flexible path sketched out ahead of time.

Have an easy answer on hand. The simple question, "So, do you have kids?" takes on a strong sense of invasiveness when you're childless against your preference. It helps to remember that the vast majority of people ask such questions innocently, in an attempt to make conversation. Having a simple answer on hand will allow you to regain control over how much people know about your infertility.

When asked if you have children, reply with true-but-not-bean-spilling phrases such as "We're working on it," or "We think about children a lot," recommends Harriet Rovner-Ferguson, C.S.W., a psychotherapist specializing in infertility in Smithtown, New York, and author of *Experiencing Infertility*. This kind of polite yet vague answer allows you to honor your need for privacy without having to be too secretive. It leaves room for you to go on to share more information—or not—as your mood and the moment dictate.

Talk yourself down. Loss of control during infertility may become so extreme that some women experience panic attacks. These unpredictable episodes of racing heartbeat, perspiration, anxiety, and fear of dying can be incredibly frightening. Learning what the attacks are is often enough to get them under control, says Hieger. Talking kindly and calmly to yourself can also help. Hieger recommends repeating phrases to yourself, such as "I understand why I'm feeling this way," or "Not everything is out of my control."

EXPAND YOUR VISION OF YOURSELF

Infertility can become an all-consuming issue, taking up most of your time and all of your energy. "What happens is that women begin to define themselves as infertile," says Rovner-Ferguson. You may find yourself identifying with your problematic reproductive organs, rather than with the rest of your body and the rest of your life.

It may be tough to remember the days when you did more than visit doctors or pine away after every baby spotted on the street. But it's crucial to your healing that you do so. If you find that thoughts about infertility are in your head every minute, the following tips can help you get back in touch with the parts of your life that you may not be tapping into.

"File a report" every day. Nurture yourself and counter negative thinking at the same time with an exercise that one expert calls the "new and good activity report." Rovner-Ferguson asks members of her support groups to do something good for themselves each week that promotes health and happiness in their lives. You can do this yourself, on a weekly or (even better) daily basis. Choose an activity such as taking a long bath or listening to a favorite piece of music. If you are feeling guilty or angry with yourself because of infertility, this self-nurturing exercise may seem hard at first. But give it a try. "You can't believe how helpful this is," says Rovner-Ferguson.

Keep the problem in perspective. Women with infertility may feel like nothing more than a defective baby-making machine. "This kind of thinking can happen with any kind of major illness," says Rovner-Ferguson. Try to keep the focus narrow by reminding yourself that only a part of your body is infertile, not your entire being. For example, she notes that when President Ronald Reagan was dealing with a serious illness, he "put it in perspective when he said something like, 'My stomach has cancer—I don't.'"

PROTECT YOUR RELATIONSHIP

It's sadly ironic. The goal of overcoming infertility is to produce a baby—the result of the loving union between two partners. But the stress of infertility can be a real drain on a couple's relationship resources, threatening the very foundation of the family you are striving so hard to build.

Other hallmarks of baby-making—that is, intimacy and sex—also suffer when a couple faces infertility, particularly if a woman is undergoing assisted reproduction procedures. "If 'sex' is happening in the doctor's office, it may not be happening at home," says Rovner-Ferguson. Even if you are not being treated medically, having to have sex on schedule, whether you are in the mood or not, can take the spark out of it. The constant worry about failure and the feelings of responsibility for each other's disappointment can all wreak havoc on even the strongest partnership.

But infertility doesn't have to do permanent damage to your union.

This crisis can be a learning opportunity—a chance to learn more about your partner's coping style, as well as a time to learn more about how to take care of each other.

Realize it's "different copes for different folks." Men and women are different in so many ways, and the experience of infertility really puts those differences under the microscope. Being aware of each other's unique coping styles can help keep you together at a time when you need each other most. "I tell my clients that the first thing to become aware of is that your spouse does not cope the same way you do," says Silvia Schneider Fox, Psy.D., a licensed clinical psychologist and director of support services for RESOLVE of Illinois in Chicago. Men are often more oriented toward problem-solving; women tend to want to vent their feelings. Expecting your mate to mirror your coping style can be very disappointing. "A woman may not be able to get exactly what she needs from her husband, and she may wind up feeling misunderstood," says Dr. Fox. A better option is to supplement the support you do receive from your partner with the support of other women who have been through infertility.

Take a time-out. When you feel like you are running a race against infertility, stepping onto the sidelines for even a short time can seem counterintuitive. But taking a break from baby-making is one of the best things you can do for your relationship, says Dr. Fox. Stopping treatment, or even going back to using birth control for a time, can give you room to breathe again. "It can help you both tune into your emotional needs and give you a chance to figure out what is important in your life as a couple," Dr. Fox says. If taking an extended break seems too scary, consider even just a weekend with no discussion of infertility or infertility treatment. Let others know you're taking a time-out, or plan a trip to a place where no one will ask questions about treatment or your next doctor appointment.

FIND STRENGTH IN SUPPORT GROUPS

Support groups can make the inherently lonely experience of infertility less isolating. In fact, support groups offer what may be the most important tool for women experiencing infertility: emotional connection with other women who are in the same situation. "You can say anything you need to in that environment and feel safe," says Hieger, who has run infertility support groups for the past 21 years.

Find the group for you. Infertility support groups come in more than one "flavor." Groups focus on issues such as stress management, relationship building, treatment options, and pregnancy loss, among others. Ask your doctor or nurse for a referral, or call your local chapter of RESOLVE: The National Infertility Association and ask for a list of available support groups. Choose the one that appeals to you most strongly; you can always switch or join another at a later time.

Share, but don't compare. Support groups offer a healthy outlet where women can share the stories of what they may be going through—including news of medical protocols, special diet or rest regimens, and other treatments. While it's helpful to talk things out, be wary of comparing your treatments or failures with those of other women, cautions George Attia, M.D., director of IVF services and head of the fertility program at the University of Texas in Dallas. "Bring your medical questions to your doctor to get the most accurate information."

CONSIDER COUNSELING

Infertility counseling is therapy when you need it most. A trained counselor can help you cope with grief and loss and teach you ways to reduce anxiety, stress, and depression. A counselor well-versed in the experience of infertility can also help couples and individuals navigate confusing choices and difficult decisions, allowing you to move ahead when you may feel stuck. An infertility counselor can be a psychiatrist, a psychologist, a social worker, a nurse, a marriage and family therapist, or even a clergy member. Be sure that any counselor you consider is licensed to practice, has a graduate degree in a mental health field, and has been trained in the medical and emotional aspects of infertility. That last requirement is particularly crucial—you want to make sure that whomever you choose to talk with understands exactly what you are going through, including any medical jargon you may have to deal with as well as specific emotional reactions you may be feeling.

While you should feel free to schedule an appointment with an infertility counselor at any time, certain signs indicate that seeing a counselor should be a priority. Just as with clinical depression, these symptoms can occur alone or in combination.

* Persistent feelings of sadness, guilt, or worthlessness

* Loss of interest in usual activities

* Agitation or anxiety

* Constant preoccupation with infertility

* Difficulty concentrating or remembering

* Change in appetite, weight, or sleep patterns

* Increased use of alcohol or drugs

* Thoughts of suicide or death

* Depression

* Increased mood swings

* Marital discord

Finding an infertility counselor is easier than you might think. You don't need to scan the yellow pages or whisper into friends' ears (although both of those approaches would probably work, too). Professional, compassionate help is as close as your medical doctor, your computer, or your telephone.

Ask your doctor for a referral. If you are seeing a medical doctor for infertility treatment, he or she can easily direct you to a qualified infertility counselor—all you have to do is ask. "I actually bring the subject up at the time of the first visit," says G. David Adamson, M.D., a reproductive endocrinologist who is director of Fertility Physicians of Northern California in San Jose and Palo Alto and clinical professor at Stanford University School of Medicine. "An infertility counselor can help people phrase any questions they may want to ask me, and also assist them in making good choices."

Call on a professional organization. A number of professional groups can refer you to an infertility counselor in your area. Organizations such as the American Society for Reproductive Medicine have member directories on their Web sites as well as helplines that provide telephone assistance. (See Resources on page 315 for contact information.)

ADOPTION: ANOTHER PATH TO PARENTING

When you discover (or remember) that your urge to parent is stronger than your dream of giving birth, you'll know that the time has come to consider adopting a child. But that's an important distinction to make, says Katherine Zieman, N.D., a naturopathic physician in Gresham, Oregon, who resolved her infertility by becoming the mother of two adopted children.

"Most people have a strong desire to have children," notes Dr. Zieman. But it's important to think further into your motivation to create a family. What is the most important part of the experience for you—to undergo the unique physical challenge of childbirth or to simply and finally be a mother? "It's when people find out they cannot have a biological child that their underlying reason for wanting a child surfaces," she says.

For women who truly crave the event of birth, medical intervention may help them achieve their goal of pregnancy. Living without parenting is another natural choice for other women who discover that the urge to give birth was stronger than their desire to parent. But if you examine your innermost feelings and find that being parents—by hook or by crook—is really the most important thing to you and your mate, adoption is a wonderful answer to your prayers. If you've been dreaming of becoming pregnant, making a conscious transition to adoption will help you move ahead with clarity and confidence. Here are some expert tips for making the psychological and spiritual shift to opening your heart to adoption.

Embrace adoption. Actively *choosing* adoption (instead of simply accepting it as the only option left to you) means that when you finally hold your new baby or child in your arms, you'll leave regret behind and look forward to the adventure of parenting. "You need to embrace adoption," says Sharon Covington, M.S.W., director of psychological support services at Shady Grove Fertility in Rockville, Maryland, and author of *Infertility Counseling*. "Accept adoption as second choice—but not second best."

Grieve the loss of the biological child who never was. Rather than playing "sour grapes" by simply turning your back on the unfulfilled desire to be pregnant and give birth, acknowledge the unrealized dream—and let yourself grieve for it. "I had to consciously let go of my desire for the experience of pregnancy and birth," says Dr. Zieman. Some women or

THE FOUR MAJOR STEPS TO ADOPTION

If you choose to pursue adoption through an agency (rather than independently), you'll have to move through four basic steps. While the details will differ in each case, here is a brief look at what generally happens. Be sure to do additional research before you get started in order to learn all you can about the adoption process as well as the choices you have.

1. Choose an adoption agency. You can select a private or public adoption agency. A private agency should be licensed by the state where it operates. Private agencies handle domestic and international adoptions and can charge thousands of dollars for their services. A public adoption agency is a branch of your state's social service agency. Public agencies usually handle only special-needs adoptions (not infants or international adoptions), and the fees are usually modest compared to private agencies.

2. Complete the application and preplacement assessment. The adoption agency you contact will ask you to fill out an application form. After being accepted by the agency, you will have to undergo a "home study" or preplacement family assessment. The home study basically evaluates couples or individuals as prospective adoptive families. You will be interviewed, probably more than once. The questions asked might seem intrusive, but it helps to remember that the study's goal is to ensure a

couples even opt to mark their time of grieving with a ceremony or symbolic ritual, such as putting together a small shrine dedicated to their unborn child or by burying or burning records of failed medical procedures.

Allow yourself to "speak" to the spirits of any lost children. The idea here is to make peace with any children you may have lost in the past—whether through miscarriages, abortions, or failed reproductive treatments. You can "talk" to the children through prayer or silent meditation. Writing a journal entry in the form of a letter is also helpful. Ask for forgiveness, if you feel the need to be forgiven. You can also ask the spirit of a past child to "find" you again by helping you in your search for a birth mother.

---

nurturing, safe home for every child placed. Prospective parents may also be required to take a physical exam and may have to undergo a background check to rule out a history of child abuse.

3. Prepare to be patient. The waiting game depends on the child you are hoping to adopt. White infants can take the longest time—up to 5 years in some cases. Prospective parents seeking an African-American infant may have a shorter wait, possibly less than 6 months. International adoptions can take a year or more. And special-needs children are always waiting for parents. Regardless of the type of adoption you pursue, after the child is found there will still be weeks or even months of waiting while final arrangements are made.

4. Make it all legal. Adoption is a complicated legal process; you'll need a lawyer to help you fulfill the legal requirements. International adoptions are usually finalized before the child leaves her birth country, although a lot depends on the type of visa your child has and the laws particular to your state. Once your child is home with you, you'll also have to naturalize her as a U.S. citizen. Domestic adoptions are usually finalized about 6 months after you've brought your child home. The agency will probably work with you during this time to provide a report to the court recommending approval of adoption. Your lawyer will then file with the court to complete the process.

Doing this kind of internal exercise can bring a surprising amount of peace to a woman's mind, says Dr. Zieman.

Once you've sorted out your feelings about the physical act of giving birth versus your pure desire to be a parent, it's time to do some serious research. Adoption, whether independent (working directly with a birth mother) or through an agency, domestic (an American child) or international (a child from another country), is a complicated process. Get all the information you can about the steps, costs, and social reactions involved so that you will be better prepared for the road ahead—the road that leads to your long-awaited child.

Attend an adoption conference or discussion. The best way to get an overview of the legal and logistical processes of adoption is to attend an adoption discussion. Since adoption laws can vary quite a bit from state to state, a local conference can also provide you with specific information on adoption where you live. Ask your doctor about upcoming discussions, or check the RESOLVE Web site for listings by area (see page 319).

Talk to other adoptive parents. Adoptive parents are often eager to talk about their children and the process it took to bring them home. Such people might also be able to offer advice or recommend specific agencies or lawyers who were particularly helpful to them. Attend an adoption support group or post a message on an adoption message board or chat room. Extend an invitation for an adoptive parent to talk with you; don't be surprised if you are inundated with positive responses.

THE SINGLE-CHILD FAMILY

You did it once before, but this time, pregnancy is frustratingly, heartbreakingly, confusingly elusive. Unlike other women with infertility who "don't know what they're missing," you *do* know—all too well.

According to RESOLVE, secondary infertility is actually more common than primary infertility. Regardless, many who are experiencing secondary infertility feel left out and unable to identify with women facing primary infertility. "I feel funny in the infertility support groups and even on the

Web sites," says Andrea Mercadente, an Amsterdam, New York, woman challenged by secondary infertility. "I feel like I don't fit in."

Couples experiencing secondary infertility also often worry about appearing ungrateful for the child they already have or greedy for another. The fact is, secondary infertility is a difficult challenge, one that requires just as much care and compassion as primary infertility.

Seek out a specialty support group. Most infertility resources are aimed at people who have no children, making it hard for couples and women experiencing secondary infertility to find the unique support they need. RESOLVE offers specialized secondary infertility support groups and can also provide referrals to therapists trained in this area of counseling. (See page 319 for contact information.)

Feel the "strength of three." While your yearnings for another child feel powerful, don't forget the strength that already exists in your family of three. There can be many pluses to having a single-child family. Focus on the love and warmth your small family shares and be sure to do fun activities together.

Share age-appropriate information with your child. Secondary infertility affects children, too. Your child may truly want a sibling—or she may wonder why you want another baby so much. Rather than tiptoeing around the subject, be as honest as you can with your child. Explain that you can't have another baby right now but that together you are all still very much a family—no matter what happens.

THE ROAD LESS TRAVELED: CHOOSING THE CHILD-FREE LIFE

When you think of a woman or couple without children, what image comes to mind? You might picture a lonely old spinster or maybe the one crotchety couple at the end of the block who frowned at anyone walking past their yard. But times are changing. The fact is, more and more people are choosing to live child-free, either as a resolution to infertility or as an alternative lifestyle choice.

Much of the difference rides on the words—and the attitudes—we use. The term "childless" implies an enforced lack or loss of something. "Child-free" includes the idea of liberty and personal choice. To live child-free, you need to turn involuntary childlessness into *voluntary* childlessness.

Try child-free on a trial basis. Unlike having or adopting a child, the child-free choice is not irreversible. Before making the decision to commit to life without parenting, you can "try on" the lifestyle for a length of time. But remember, it takes a real attitude shift to switch gears from yearning for a child to being positive about living child-free—you shouldn't simply squelch your desires for a child. An infertility counselor or child-free (sometimes referred to as "living without parenting") support group or on-line chat community can help you make a healthy adjustment to your thinking.

Go back to birth control. While you and your mate are trying out the child-free life, and once you have made the decision to choose this path, it's a good idea to go back to birth control—as strange as that may seem or feel. Eliminating the possibility of pregnancy, as well as the potential monthly disappointment of not conceiving, will free you and your mate from the cycle of raised and dashed hopes. You may also find that using birth control gives you a peace of mind you may not have expected. About 2 years after Sue Slotnick and her husband made the conscious decision not to parent, her period was late. "I immediately thought to myself, 'Oh, no!'" recalls Slotnick. The false alarm offered her an interesting insight. "It became very clear to me then that living without parenting is the best choice for me."

Continue to nurture. Living child-free can actually be seen as a gift to the people around you, says Gina Burns, a San Francisco woman who has undergone treatment for infertility; she and her husband are now leaning toward the child-free lifestyle. "There is a tremendous opportunity for people without children to find other outlets for their nurturing instincts," says Burns. Spend your loving energy on friends and family; you could also volunteer to work with children, seniors, or animals.

PART FIVE

CHECKLISTS
FOR
ACTION

WHAT TO DO 1 TO 20 YEARS BEFORE TRYING

First step: Assess your "real" reproductive age (see page 26).

MEDICAL STEPS

❑ Get an annual gynecological exam, including Pap test, pelvic exam, and screenings for sexually transmitted diseases (STDs).

❑ Schedule an annual physical.

❑ Get biannual dental exams.

❑ Get mammograms starting at age 35 or earlier depending on family history.

❑ Have a thyroid screening beginning at age 35 or if you experience symptoms of thyroid problems (see page 249).

❑ Be conservative about getting x-rays, which subject eggs to radiation.

❑ Pursue fertility-preserving steps if you need cancer treatment, as described on page 159.

LIFESTYLE FACTORS

❑ Resolve any substance abuse problems.

❑ Maintain your weight at no more than 15 percent above or below your ideal body mass index, as defined on page 82.

❑ If new to fitness, begin walking 20 to 30 minutes several times a week.

❑ Reduce sugar, caffeine, saturated fats, and processed and fast food in your diet.

❑ Increase consumption of organic fruits and vegetables and whole grains.

❑ Practice "safe sex" by using a condom every time you have sex.

❑ Aggressively avoid exposure to pesticides, radiation, heavy metals, solvents, and even toxins in common household products, as described in chapter 9.

❑ Filter your drinking and bathing water (see chapter 9).

EMOTIONAL MAINTENANCE

❑ Discuss childbearing intentions with your potential mate.

❑ Seek psychological counseling for issues of previous loss, esteem problems, history of abuse, or mental health concerns.

❑ Practice a daily relaxation technique.

❑ Evaluate whether your career is mentally and physically sustaining or leaves you feeling burned-out.

❑ Evaluate your financial plan with your partner, and adjust for child-raising considerations.

INFORMATION TO GET

❑ Check your family history of menopause to help gauge the length of your reproductive years.

❑ Discuss reproductive and sexual histories with your potential mate.

❑ Ask your health care practitioner if your current medications and nutritional supplements are safe for use during pregnancy so you can begin to substitute for or phase out those that aren't.

IF YOU WANT TO GO THE EXTRA STEP

❑ Set up early preconception counseling with an ob/gyn, family doctor, or nurse-midwife.

❑ Keep a week-long food journal and have it evaluated by a registered dietitian.

❑ In addition to increasing your selections of organic food, make vegetarian meals and raw foods part of your diet.

❑ Have baseline tests of follicle-stimulating hormone (FSH) and inhibin taken to estimate how close you are to perimenopause.

❑ Switch to feminine hygiene products that aren't chlorine-bleached (see chapter 9).

WHAT TO DO 1 TO 12 MONTHS BEFORE TRYING

First step: Work on anything listed above that you haven't done yet, and get a preconception care screening with a health care practitioner or educator particularly experienced in preconception care.

MEDICAL STEPS

❑ Schedule a preconception counseling visit with your gynecologist, family doctor, or midwife 6 months before trying.

❑ Get a complete physical, including standard blood and urine tests, and any immunizations you and your doctor feel are necessary (be aware that after getting certain vaccinations, you'll need to wait 1 to 3 months before trying to conceive).

❑ Get a careful evaluation of any menstrual, hormonal, or sexual problems during your annual ob–gyn exam.

❑ Make sure any STDs and pregnancy-threatening infections you had in the past have been effectively treated.

❑ After the age of 35, get an FSH–estradiol test to estimate how close you are to perimenopause.

LIFESTYLE FACTORS

❑ Start taking a daily prenatal multivitamin and mineral supplement.

❑ Consider additional supplements such as fish or flax oil, probiotics, and "green foods."

❑ Maintain a fitness program.

❑ Continue using birth control until you're cleared as "pregnancy ready" by your health care practitioner.

❑ Once cleared, switch to a natural family planning method of birth control, as described in chapter 12.

EMOTIONAL MAINTENANCE

❑ Evaluate your communications dynamic with your partner, and seek counseling if necessary (see chapter 7).

❑ Have an ongoing discussion with your partner about lifestyle changes you both will need to make for parenthood (see chapter 7).

❑ Discuss parenting roles and expectations with your partner.

❑ Spend time with children of all ages to get a sense of parenting demands and styles.

INFORMATION TO GET

❑ Find out how long it takes for cycles to normalize after quitting your birth control method.

❑ Investigate your options for pregnancy caretakers in your area, including obstetrician/gynecologists, midwives, nurse-practitioners, and family doctors.

❑ Weigh both pros and cons of common prepregnancy vaccinations such as measles–mumps–rubella, hepatitis, and chickenpox (see chapter 10).

❑ Investigate preconception, prenatal, and perinatal medical insurance coverage.

❑ Investigate your employers' maternity leave policy.

❑ Explore child care options.

IF YOU WANT TO GO THE EXTRA STEP

❑ Seek counseling with a genetics expert, particularly if you are over 35 or have any family history of birth defects or genetic illness.

❑ Work with an environmental medicine expert to overcome toxic exposures, hidden allergies, and nutritional imbalances.

❑ Develop an ephistogram (see "Fertility Visionaries" on page 108) to identify familial patterns you and your partner might want to reinforce or break away from in preparation for parenthood.

AS YOU'RE TRYING TO CONCEIVE

First step: In addition to anything above you haven't yet done, zero in on an ovulation awareness method that suits your personality and lifestyle. (see chapter 12).

MEDICAL STEPS

❑ If you were recently vaccinated, consider waiting 1 to 3 months before trying to conceive.

❑ Avoid getting run-down, since fevers and low immunity can hamper ovulation.

❑ If fertility awareness methods indicate that you haven't ovulated for two or more cycles, or if you experience irregular cycles, see your gynecologist or fertility specialist immediately.

LIFESTYLE FACTORS

❑ Zero in on your favorite ovulation awareness method, as described in chapter 12.

❑ Abstain from alcohol, or limit your consumption to less than five drinks per week.

❑ Abstain from or limit caffeine consumption to less than 250 milligrams per day (no more than two cups of coffee).

❑ Continue to aggressively avoid exposure to pesticides, radiation, heavy metals, solvents, and other chemicals.

❑ Continue taking daily prenatal multivitamin and mineral supplements.

❑ Protect yourself from toxoplasmosis infection by avoiding the following: cat litter, gardening near animal feces, and eating undercooked meat.

❑ To maintain normal ovulation, optimize sleep habits, light exposure, stress management, and other issues elaborated on in chapters 14 and 16.

EMOTIONAL MAINTENANCE

- ❏ Check in with a therapist about any fears or concerns related to childbearing.

- ❏ Keep pressure and staleness out of lovemaking with the techniques described on pages 196 to 201.

- ❏ Write or draw in a journal to support self-realization processes and to express concerns.

INFORMATION TO GET

- ❏ Ask for an infertility workup if you or your partner experienced fertility problems or if you've had a miscarriage in the past.

- ❏ Arm yourself with ovulation-detecting tools such as natural family planning charts and CycleBeads (see chapter 12).

IF YOU WANT TO GO THE EXTRA STEP

- ❏ Consult a professional fertility awareness educator to enhance your ovulation timing.

- ❏ Take cough syrup (but not products containing antihistamines) to enhance cervical secretions (see chapter 13).

IF 6 TO 12 MONTHS HAVE GONE BY WITH NO SUCCESS

First step: Schedule appointments for both you and your partner with your family doctor, obstetrician/gynecologist, urologist, or infertility specialist for a basic fertility evaluation.

MEDICAL STEPS

❑ Pursue a basic infertility evaluation, including standard lab tests and imaging diagnostics (described in chapter 15).

❑ Ask for a prescription for progesterone if you are over 35 or taking clomiphene citrate (Clomid).

❑ With your partner and doctor, draft a long-term treatment plan, deciding in advance how much time and money you can commit to various treatment options.

❑ Get bodywork (massage, Rolfing) to improve structural abnormalities and decrease stress.

LIFESTYLE FACTORS

❑ Tone down overzealous exercise so that you're running less than 10 miles a week and biking less than 50 miles a week.

❑ Follow a detoxification regimen, including a minifast and colon cleansing, as outlined on pages 237 to 240.

❑ Practice at least 20 minutes of a relaxation technique daily, and give yourself at least one self-nurture "gift" a week (a massage, a long nap, the afternoon off, and so on).

EMOTIONAL MAINTENANCE

❑ Continue to explore concerns and self-realizations in your journal.

❑ Explore fertility-enriching meditations and visualizations (described in chapter 18).

❑ Challenge self-defeating thoughts that could suppress your life-giving energy (see chapters 6 and 18).

- ❑ Consider joining a support group like RESOLVE: The National Infertility Association (see chapter 19).
- ❑ Periodically take a break from baby-making for one or more cycles.

INFORMATION TO GET

- ❑ Understand the pros and cons of surgical interventions for structural problems like endometriosis and fibroids.
- ❑ Understand the pros and cons of fertility drugs (see chapters 15 and 16).
- ❑ Collect information on various adoption agencies and procedures.

IF YOU WANT TO GO THE EXTRA STEP

- ❑ In addition to standard lab tests, get your insulin levels tested.
- ❑ Consider acupuncture to help treat underlying hormonal and nutritional imbalances.
- ❑ Seek out a professional infertility counselor to help you make decisions and cope with grief or relationship stressors.

PRECONCEPTION CARE FOR MEN

First step: Become familiar with toxic substances you work with in your job and hobbies, and make every effort to avoid exposure.

MEDICAL STEPS

❑ Perform a monthly testicular self-exam (see chapter 2).

❑ See a urologist about any concerns with pelvic organs or sex life.

❑ If you need chemotherapy, radiation, or pelvic surgery, consider sperm preservation (see chapter 10).

LIFESTYLE FACTORS

❑ Resolve substance abuse, including marijuana use (which is sperm-inhibiting).

❑ When working with any potentially hazardous chemical, follow universal safety precautions (frequent handwashing, proper ventilation, protective equipment).

❑ If you work with toxic substances, leave your clothes, shoes, and equipment at the work site and shower before you get home.

❑ Cut out androgenic steroids and other bodybuilding supplements unless approved by a doctor.

❑ Wear a cup and other protective sports equipment.

❑ Maintain your weight at no more than 15 percent above or below your ideal body mass index, as described on page 82.

EMOTIONAL MAINTENANCE

❑ Discuss childbearing expectations with your potential mate.

❑ Evaluate your communications dynamic with your partner, and seek counseling if necessary (see chapter 7).

❑ Discuss parenting roles and expectations with your partner.

❑ Spend time with children of all ages to get a sense of parenting demands and styles.

❑ Prepare physical space for a baby in your home.

❑ Evaluate your financial plan with your partner, and adjust for child-raising considerations.

INFORMATION TO GET

❑ Check reproductive health hazards for all the chemicals you work with in your job or hobby by consulting the relevant material safety data sheets and a teratogen information service (see chapter 9).

❑ Ask your health care practitioner if your current medications (even over the counter) and nutritional supplements are safe for conception so you can phase them out in advance if they're not.

❑ Investigate your employers' family leave policies and, if necessary, push for better provisions.

❑ Investigate preconception, prenatal, and perinatal medical insurance coverage.

IF YOU WANT TO GO THE EXTRA STEP

❑ Have a baseline semen analysis taken before you try to conceive.

❑ Have your home's radiation levels tested, paying particular attention to the bedroom.

STEPS FOR MEN TRYING TO BECOME FATHERS

First step: Have a semen analysis done if you and your partner haven't had success in 12 months, or in 6 months if she is 35 or older.

MEDICAL STEPS

- ❑ If you haven't conceived in 6 to 12 months, have at least two semen analyses performed (3 to 4 weeks apart).

- ❑ To help improve low or abnormal sperm counts, consider supplements of *Panax ginseng* and Pycnogenol (see chapter 16 for dosages).

- ❑ If hormone deficiencies are compromising your fertility, follow the detoxification regimen, including a minifast and colon cleansing, outlined on pages 237 to 240.

LIFESTYLE FACTORS

- ❑ Avoid steam rooms and long soaks in the tub while attempting conception and 3 months in advance.

- ❑ Take hourly breaks during car rides and bike rides (to avoid overheating sperm or impeding penile bloodflow).

- ❑ Be more aggressive than ever to avoid pesticides, radiation, heavy metals, solvents, and other chemicals described in chapters 9 and 14.

- ❑ Take a high-quality daily multivitamin/mineral supplement for men, or individual B vitamins and antioxidants recommended on page 66.

EMOTIONAL MAINTENANCE

- ❑ Fend off the baby-making stress of lovemaking with the techniques described on pages 196 to 201.

- ❑ Make foreplay a priority with your partner during conception attempts (see chapter 13).

- ❑ Make every effort to "hear out" your mate's concerns and frustrations with infertility, and be sure to share your own.

INFORMATION TO GET

❑ Find out if your fertility odds could be enhanced with surgical intervention for a structural abnormality, such as varicocele or hypospadias.

❑ Find out if fertility odds could be enhanced with fertility drugs to correct hormone deficiencies.

❑ If you have a serious sperm deficiency, see if you are a candidate for sperm retrieval or the intracytoplasmic sperm injection techniques featured in chapter 15.

IF YOU WANT TO GO THE EXTRA STEP

❑ While attempting conception, practice selective ejaculation (no more than every 2 to 3 days) to optimize sperm count (see chapter 13).

❑ Switch from briefs to boxer shorts and avoid tight pants in consideration of spermatic temperature sensitivity.

PART SIX
RESOURCES

Helpful Organizations

The following pages offer a range of national and international organizations that can offer additional advice, support, and referrals on topics including preconception care, environmental hazards, complementary medicine, pregnancy, and adoption.

ADOPTION

The National Adoption Information Clearinghouse (NAIC)
330 C Street, SW
Washington, DC 20447
Phone: (703) 352-3488 or (888) 251-0075
Fax: (703) 385-3206
www.calib.com/naic
Sponsored by the Department of Health and Human Services, NAIC can connect you with state agencies, legal services, and adoption support groups throughout the United States. To access their National Adoption Search Directory, go to www.calib.com/naic/database/nadd/naddsearch.cfm. This organization also offers an excellent schedule of nationwide seminars on domestic and international adoptions.

COMPLEMENTARY MEDICINE

American Academy of Acupuncture and Oriental Medicine (AAAOM)

1925 West County Road B2

Roseville, MN 55113

Phone: (651) 631-0204

www.AAAOM.org

The "TCM for Common Health Problems" portion of the organization's Web site explains how Chinese medicine can enhance fertility and resolve reproductive health problems through specific dietary modifications, herbal prescriptions, stress-reduction techniques, and acupuncture treatments. Contact the AAAOM if you need help locating a practitioner in your area trained in Traditional Chinese Medicine.

American Academy of Environmental Medicine (AAEM)

7701 East Kellogg, Suite 625

Wichita, KS 67207

Phone: (316) 684-5500

Fax: (316) 684-5709

www.AAEM.com

The AAEM is a medical society of physicians from various specialties who received additional training in the prevention and treatment of environmentally triggered illnesses. The organization can refer you to physicians who have successfully completed their core curriculum.

The American Holistic Medical Association (AHMA)

12101 Menaul Boulevard, NE, Suite C

Albuquerque, NM 87112

Phone: (505) 292-7788

www.holisticmedicine.org

For $15, this organization can send you a list of medical doctors and osteopaths trained in holistic methods.

INFERTILITY SUPPORT AND PRECONCEPTION CARE

Advanced Reproductive Care, Inc. (ARC)

540 University Avenue, Suite 250

Palo Alto, CA 94301

www.arcfertility.com

ARC is a national network of physicians specializing in infertility. Nearly one-third of the nation's 700 reproductive endocrinologists participate. ARC even offers a money-back plan that refunds the treatment costs if the couple doesn't successfully conceive.

The American Infertility Association (AIA)

666 Fifth Avenue, Suite 278

New York, NY 10103

Phone: (888) 917-3777

www.americaninfertility.org

This national organization is dedicated to assisting women and men facing decisions related to family building and reproductive health. AIA offers a free information packet, including fact sheets and brochures covering many topics related to infertility and adoption. It also sponsors an annual infertility and adoption conference geared toward the patient. Those who join AIA can attend weekly support groups led by trained therapists.

The Center for Creative Parenting

PO Box 2024

Petaluma, CA 94952

Phone: (707) 781-3438

www.creativeparenting.com

Harvard-trained holistic counselor Carista Luminare-Rosen, Ph.D., has two areas of expertise: educating potential parents to prepare mentally, spiritually, and physically for the role of parenting and interfacing with Eastern and Western doctors to guide couples with fertility challenges through treatment. Contact the Center to find out more about her classes, workshops, telephone consultations, newsletters, media appearances, and audiotapes.

Foresight: The Association for the Promotion of Preconceptual Care
28 The Paddock
Godalming, Surrey, England GU7 1XD
Phone: 011-44-1483-427839
Fax: 011-44-1483-427668
www.foresight-preconception.org.uk
For more than 30 years, this organization has helped thousands of couples worldwide have exceptionally healthy pregnancies and children. Its prime focus is on avoiding environmental toxins and optimizing nutrition. Foresight has a wealth of books and pamphlets to guide men and women in optimizing their physical readiness for conception. To get further information, enclose a self-addressed, stamped envelope with your request and mail to the address above, or visit the organization's Web site.

The InterNational Council on Infertility Information Dissemination, Inc. (INCIID)
PO Box 6836
Arlington, VA 22206
Phone: (703) 379-9178
www.inciid.org
Formed by three women who overcame infertility, this organization boasts members from all continents and a strong board of medical advisors who provide online fact sheets and articles to couples facing infertility and loss.

Mothers 35 Plus
www.mothers35plus.co.uk
Originally developed as an over-35 mother's college project, this U.K.-based Web site has become a source for anecdotal information and support for older mothers worldwide.

RESOLVE: The National Infertility Association
1310 Broadway
Somerville, MA 02144
Helpline: (888) 623-0774
www.resolve.org
Since 1974, RESOLVE has provided education, advocacy, and emotional support to men and women who struggle with infertility. In addition to its physician referral service and Web resources, each chapter in their nationwide network offers support group meetings.

OCCUPATIONAL HEALTH

Occupational Safety and Health Administration (OSHA)
200 Constitution Avenue, NW
Washington, DC 20210
(800) 321-OSHA (6742)
www.osha.gov
Contact this government agency to file a complaint related to hazardous conditions on your job (you can do it online) or find more information about work-related hazards.

Organization of Teratology Information Services (OTIS)
National referral number: (866) 626-6847
This national organization can refer you to the reproductive health authority in your state who is trained to answer questions on the effects of specific drugs, medications, and chemicals on a pregnancy or potential pregnancy.

PREGNANCY AND CHILD HEALTH

The Association of Prenatal and Perinatal Psychology and Health (APPPAH)
PO Box 1398
Forestville, CA 95436
Phone: (707) 857-4041

This educational organization is dedicated to exploring the physical, emotional, mental, and spiritual development and health of the unborn and newborn child.

March of Dimes
2700 South Quincy Street, Suite 220
Arlington, VA 22206
Phone: (888) MODIMES
www.modimes.org

Founded by President Franklin D. Roosevelt in the 1930s, the March of Dimes has helped to save the lives of millions of babies. As leading sources of information on the prevention of birth defects, their specialists are eager to answer your questions by phone, e-mail, or online chat.

National Women's Health Information Center
Phone: (800) 994-WOMAN or (800) 994-9662
TDD: (888) 220-5446
www.4women.gov

This Department of Health and Human Services organization features a "healthy pregnancy" link on its Web site. You'll find interactive tools such as a quiz to test your knowledge of pregnancy, an ovulation calculator, and a due date calculator.

REPRODUCTIVE HEALTH

The American Society for Reproductive Medicine (ASRM)
1209 Montgomery Highway
Birmingham, AL 35216-2809
Phone: (205) 978-5000
www.asrm.org

Originally known as the American Fertility Society, the ASRM has brought fertility experts together since 1944 to further the field of reproductive health. Members include obstetrician/gynecologists, urologists, reproductive endocrinologists, embryologists, mental health professionals, internists, nurses, practice administrators, laboratory technicians, pediatricians, research scientists, and veterinarians. The ASRM Patient Education Committee produces booklets and patient fact sheets that can help you navigate the complexities of various reproductive disorders and their treatment. The organization also offers referrals to practitioners.

American Urological Association
1120 North Charles Street
Baltimore, MD 21201
Phone: (410) 727-1100
Fax: (410) 223-4370
www.auanet.org
This educational, nonprofit organization claims to be the world's preeminent urological association, with more than 13,000 members. Contact it for information on genitourinary conditions.

Association of Reproductive Health Professionals (ARHP)
2401 Pennsylvania Avenue, Suite 350
Washington, DC 20037-1718
www.arhp.org
This nonprofit national medical organization has been educating providers and their patients since 1963 about important reproductive health issues, including contraception, sexually transmitted diseases, HIV/AIDS, menopause, urogenital infections, cancer prevention and detection, abortion, sexuality, and infertility.

Endometriosis Association (EA)
8585 North 76th Place
Milwaukee, WI 53223
Phone: (800) 992-ENDO
www.endometriosisassn.org
Through its Web site and newsletter, this compassionate nonprofit group can provide you with basic educational materials, as well as ongoing updates on endometriosis research and treatment options. The association

also maintains a directory of physicians who specialize in the disease and organizes support groups throughout the country.

Hysterectomy Educational Resources and Services Foundation (HERS)

422 Bryn Mawr Avenue
Bala Cynwyd, PA 19004
Phone: (888) 750-HERS

This independent, nonprofit, international women's health education organization provides information about hysterectomy, its adverse effects, and alternative treatments. Its many services include telephone counseling and a comprehensive list of books and medical research that can help you make a well-informed decision about surgery of the reproductive organs.

Polycystic Ovarian Syndrome Association (PCOSA)

PO Box 80517
Portland, OR 97280
Phone: (877) 775-PCOS
www.pcosupport.org

Contact this nonprofit group to learn more about its wealth of support groups, online discussions, and educational resources. In addition to providing general diet and lifestyle advice, the organization posts articles by syndrome experts specifically for women trying to conceive and features stories about successful pregnancies.

The Prostatitis Foundation

1063 30th Street, Box 8
Smithshire, IL 61478
Phone: (888) 891-4200
www.prostatitis.org

This organization is a source of hope for men who have not been able to achieve relief from chronic prostate infections with conventional treatment. The Web site and newsletter fuse personal anecdotes and the guidance of prostatitis experts to show how men can physically and emotionally heal from this insidious condition.

Environmentally Friendly Companies

These companies are known for their commitment to providing products that are nontoxic and environmentally sound. While this list is not meant to be comprehensive, it does offer a good starting point for locating everything from organically grown food to chlorine-free feminine hygiene products to nontoxic household cleaners and laundry products.

American Formulating and Manufacturing (AFM)

Phone: (800) 239-0321

www.afmsafecoat.com

AFM claims to be the only company to provide a complete range of chemically responsible building and maintenance products. They supply the Safecoat and SafeChoice brands of environmentally sensitive paint, primers, stains, and finishing products, as well as industrial carpet cleaners and sealants approved by environmental medicine physicians.

Body Elements/Terressentials

2220 North 3rd Street

Arlington, VA 22201-1712

Phone: (703) 525-0585

This company is recommended by the Endometriosis Association as a good source for safe feminine hygiene products, including chlorine-free tampons and washable pads.

Lehman's Non-Electric Catalog

One Lehman Circle

PO Box 41

Kidron, OH 44636

Phone: (877) GET LEHMANS or (877) 438-5346

Fax: (888) 780-4975 or (330) 857-5785

E-mail: info@Lehmans.com

www.lehmans.com

Lehman's offers more than 3,000 products for simple, healthy living with an emphasis on nonelectric items (to cut down on your radiation exposure). Some examples are hand-powered tools, solar merchandise, and ingenious gadgets to process your homegrown food.

Planet Natural

1612 Gold Avenue

Bozeman, MT 59715

Phone: (800) 289-6656 or (406) 587-5891

www.planetnatural.com

Through this catalog, you can purchase everything from nontoxic soaps and cleaning supplies to natural pest repellants and a nonpolluting lawnmower.

Seventh Generation

212 Battery Street, Suite A

Burlington, VT 05401-5281

Phone: (800) 456-1191

www.seventhgeneration.com

Self-labeled the world's most trusted brand of authentic, safe, and environmentally responsible products for a healthy home, Seventh Generation offers a full line of laundry products, household cleaners, and paper towels, bath tissue, and facial tissue that are not bleached with chlorine (they're also 100 percent recycled). You can purchase Seventh Generation products by calling its toll-free number or searching its Web site to locate a local store that stocks its goods.

SunOrganic Farm

Box 2429
Valley Center, CA 92082
(888) 269-9888
www.sunorganic.com

SunOrganic supplies a wide variety of natural home, beauty, and food products, including dioxin-free feminine hygiene products and plenty of organic grains and canned vegetables.

Whole Foods Market, Inc.

601 North Lamar, Suite 300
Austin, TX 78703
Phone: (512) 477-4455 (corporate office)
www.wholefoodsmarket.com

This national chain of health-conscious grocery stores is committed to providing organically grown foods and nontoxic products. Check with their corporate office or on their Web site to see if there's a market near you.

Wild Oats Markets, Inc.

3375 Mitchell Lane
Boulder, CO 80301
Phone: (800) 494-WILD or (800) 494-9453
www.wildoats.com

This nationwide chain of natural and organic food markets in the United States and Canada stocks the organic foods, nutritional supplements, and nontoxic products recommended by experts throughout this book. You can search their Web site to see if there's a store in your area.

Recommended Reading

Barbieri, Robert L., Alice D. Domar, and Kevin R. Loughlin. *Six Steps to Increased Fertility: An Integrated Medical and Mind/Body Approach to Promote Conception*. New York: Simon & Schuster, 2000.

The authors discuss medical interventions for infertility and explain how women can adopt the cognitive–behavioral breakthroughs of Harvard's Mind/Body Medical Institute.

The Boston Women's Health Book Collective. *Our Bodies, Ourselves for the New Millennium*. New York: Simon & Schuster, 1998.

This resource is packed with frank, inspiring discussions on childbearing decisions and sexuality through various stages of life. A guiding light to women of all walks of life since the women's revolution, this classic text is updated to include current issues, explain the latest medical procedures, and provide solid resources.

Corsello, Serafina. *The Ageless Woman*. New York: Corsello Communications, 1999.

Dr. Corsello offers strategies for vitality and longevity as well as lots of specifics on natural hormone balance through various life stages.

Hanson, Rick, Jan Hanson, and Ricki Pollycove. *Mother Nurture: A Mother's Guide to Health in Body, Mind, and Intimate Relationships.* London: Penguin, 2002.

In this book geared toward overworked moms, a well-rounded team of experts offers practical dietary, self-care, and co-parenting strategies. They also run an inspiring, interactive Web site at www.nurturemom.com

Indichova, Julia. *Inconceivable: A Woman's Triumph over Despair and Statistics.* New York: Broadway Books, 2001.

This is the personal success story of an author who achieved pregnancy at the age of 44, after revamping her diet and sense of self.

Kamhi, Ellen. *Cycles of Life: Herbs and Energy Techniques for the Stages of a Woman's Life.* New York: M. Evans, 2001.

Dr. Kamhi, a natural-health authority, offers insights into developing a more intimate relationship with one's body by discovering the beauty and joy of true self-care. This book is especially useful for women who always wanted to make their own plant medicines.

Luminare-Rosen, Carista. *Parenting Begins before Conception: A Guide to Preparing Body, Mind, and Spirit for You and Your Future Child.* Rochester: Healing Arts Press, 2000.

Dr. Luminare-Rosen offers an in-depth approach to being the most enlightened person you can for the journey of parenthood. Her self-tests, journal exercises, affirmations, and stunning insights help bring forth the best of what's inside of you.

McGee, Charles T., and Effie Poy Yew Chow. *Miracle Healing from China—Qigong.* Medipress, 1996.

This book offers Traditional Chinese Medicine techniques that can increase a person's "vital life force" in order to prevent disease and recover from serious imbalances. The authors carefully explain delightful daily exercises that they recommend for any couple hoping to conceive.

Naish, Francesca, and Janette Roberts. *Healthy Parents, Better Babies: A Couple's Guide to Natural Preconception Health Care.* Berkeley, CA: Crossing Press, 1999.

A premier Australian naturopathic doctor and a nutritionist define all the preconception guidelines that have helped thousands of their patients, including those who were previously unable to conceive. Includes every detail of ovulation prediction, including the more obscure observance of lunar cycle.

Payne, Niravi B., and Brenda Lane Richardson. *The Whole Person Fertility Program: A Revolutionary Mind-Body Program to Help You Conceive.* New York: Three Rivers Press, 1997.

A seasoned counselor gently leads you to face fears and wounds related to your culture, upbringing, and subconscious mind. Meditations, writing explorations, and visualizations help you clear any internal barriers to pregnancy.

Reiss, Fern. *The Infertility Diet: Get Pregnant and Prevent Miscarriage.* Newton, MA: Peanut Butter and Jelly Press, 1999.

Applauded by the American Society for Reproductive Medicine, this book includes recipes and food choices that the author attributes to helping her overcome secondary infertility.

Verny, Thomas. *The Secret Life of the Unborn Child.* New York: Delta, 1994.

In this classic prenatal psychology book, Dr. Verny illuminates how a child can be shaped by emotional experiences while still in the womb. The book also serves as a reminder for parents-to-be to optimize their mental health and communications dynamics before they conceive.

Weschler, Toni. *Taking Charge of Your Fertility: The Definitive Guide to Natural Birth Control, Pregnancy Achievement, and Reproductive Health.* New York: Quill, 2001.

This book is a complete primer on reading the fertility signs that empower a couple to accurately time intercourse. Includes easy-to-understand explanations of the reproductive system and a section on influencing the gender of your child.

OG magazine

Coming from a 60-year tradition of gardening in harmony with nature, OG offers focused advice for both new and seasoned organic gardeners. You can subscribe or request a free trial issue by logging on to www. organicgardening.com or call Rodale Inc. at (800) 666-2206.

Organic Style magazine

This eye-catching publication celebrates life enriched with all things organic: fashion, food, home, health, garden, travel, work, family, and soul. There are numerous resources in every issue for creating a less-toxic home without compromising luxury or beauty. To subscribe or to order a free trial issue, visit the Web site www.organicstyle.com or call Rodale Inc. at (800) 666-2206.

Index

Underscored page references indicate sidebars and tables. **Boldface** references indicate illustrations.

B

D

Daikon radish, for increasing fertility, 267
Dairy products
    allergies to, 57
    in fertility-enhancing diet, 56
    reducing consumption of, 266–67
D & C, adhesions from, 153
Dandelion
    for detoxification, 239
    safety of, 68
DBCP, affecting male fertility, 126
Deep breathing
    for body alignment, 268
    for stress reduction, 97
Dental care, preconception, 168
Depleted mother syndrome, 284–85
Depo-Provera, fertility benefits and risks
        from, 116
Depression
    help for, 171
    infertility and, 93–94, 111
DES, in beef production, 130
Desiccated thyroid supplements, 250
Detoxification
    for estrogen dominance, 249
    for hormone disorders, 237–38
    methods of, 238–40
Detoxifying Vegetable Soup, 238
Diabetes
    affecting fertility, 148–49
    gestational, 29, 148, 168
Diaphragm, for contraception, 121–22
Diet
    fertility-enhancing
        blood sugar control in, 59–61
        foods to avoid in, 57, 58, 59, 61–62
        low-glycemic foods in, 13
        natural foods in, 52–57, 61
        personal story about, 52–53
        serving sizes in, 55
    for fighting yeast overgrowth, 245–46
    as hysterectomy alternative, 35
    low-carb, for weight loss, 252–53
    for preventing prostate cancer, 45
Dioxins, as environmental hazards,
        131–32
Distress, infertility and, 93–94
Doctors, for infertility treatments, 217,
        229
Domar, Alice, 98–99

Donor eggs
    counseling about, 31
    after nonradical hysterectomy, 36
    for over-40 women, 31
Donor sperm, for male infertility, 223
Douching, avoiding, 196
Down's syndrome, incidence of, 24
Drugs. See also specific drugs
    fertility
        Clomid (see Clomiphene citrate)
        function of, 10
        health risks from, 231
        natural alternatives to, 236
        personal story about, 235–36
        side effects of, 232, 235, 236
        types of, 232
    illegal, 79, 171
    prescription and over-the-counter, 79,
        150–52
Dry brushing, for detoxification, 239–40
Dry cleaning, toxins from, 141–42
Dysfunctional uterine bleeding (DUB),
        32–33, 36

E

Early perimenopausal stage, 29–30
Early reproductive stage, 27
Eating disorders, 86, 110, 149
Echinacea, safety of, 68
Ectopic pregnancy, 231, 258
EFAs. See Essential fatty acids
Egg(s)
    chromosomal defects in, 23–24
    decline in, 21–23
    fertilization of, 20
Ejaculation
    retrograde, 261
    selective, 195
Electromagnetic fields (EMFs), reducing
        exposure to, 209–12
Embryo cryopreservation, before cancer
        treatment, 160
Embryos
    chromosomally abnormal, 23
    early development of, 21
EMFs, reducing exposure to, 209–12
Emotional baggage, releasing, 281–83
Endocrine-disrupting chemicals, affecting
        fertility, 125

F

T

U

V

Vaccinations, 158, 170
Vagina, **18**
  lubricating, 193
  maintaining health of, 195
Vaginal dryness, in late reproductive stage, 28
Vaginal ring, for contraception, 119
Varicoceles
  detection of, 44
  hydrotherapy for, 265
  male infertility from, _223_, _261_
  overheating and, 207–8
  surgery for, 257
Vas deferens, _40_, 40, 258, _261_
Vasectomy, reversing, _120–21_
Vasovasostomy, 258
Vegetables, in fertility-enhancing diet, 54–55
Visualization, fertility-enriching, 277, 282
Vitamin A, for enhancing fertility, 65
Vitamin B$_6$
  for enhancing fertility, 63
  for progesterone deficiency, 248
Vitamin B$_{12}$, for enhancing fertility, 63
Vitamin C, for enhancing fertility, 63, 65, 66–67
Vitamin E
  for enhancing fertility, 65, 67
  for preventing prostate cancer, 45
  for reducing adhesions, 259–60
Vitamins and minerals. _See also specific vitamins and minerals_
  Dietary Reference Intakes of, 63
  in multivitamins, 62–63, 66
Vitex, for regulating menstrual cycle, 29, 243
Volatile organic compounds (VOCs), as environmental hazards, 129–30

W

Wait and watch, as hysterectomy alternative, _34–35_
Water, in fertility-enhancing diet, 57, 267
Water filters, 140

Water quality, tracking, 146
Weight
  fertility and, 9, _60_, 82–83, 86–87
  ideal, determining, 82
Weight loss, with low-carb diet, _252–53_
Wheat allergy, 57, 59
Whole foods, in fertility-enhancing diet, 53–54
Whole Foods Market, Inc., 325
Whole grains, in fertility-enhancing diet, 54
Whole Person Fertility Program, The, _108–9_
Wild Oats Community Markets, Inc., 325
Wood products, safe use of, 141
Workplace
  environmental hazards in, 134–37
  radiation exposure in, 211
Wurn, Belinda, _262–63_
Wurn, Larry, _262–63_
WURN technique, _263_

X

Xenoestrogens, 249

Y

Yeast, candidiasis and, 244–46
Yeast infections, in late reproductive stage, 28
Yoga
  for infertility, 269–70, **269**
  tantric, 198
  for thyroid function, 250, **251**
Yohimbe, as aphrodisiac, _20_

Z

ZIFT. _See_ Zygote intrafallopian tube transfer
Zinc, for enhancing fertility, 65, 67, 254
Zygote intrafallopian tube transfer (ZIFT)
  procedure for, 234
  risks from, _231_